Anatomy and phys of the peripheral hearing mechanism

J. Donald Harris

THE BOBBS-MERRILL COMPANY, INC.
Indianapolis   New York

The Bobbs-Merrill
studies in
communicative
disorders

Series editor
HARVEY HALPERN

Consultant of speech-communication
RUSSELL WINDES

Copyright © 1974 by the Bobbs-Merrill Company, Inc.
Printed in the United States of America
First Printing

Library of Congress Cataloging in Publication Data
Harris, John Donald, 1914–
  Anatomy and physiology of the peripheral hearing mechanism.
  (The Bobbs-Merrill studies in communicative disorders)
  Bibliography: p.
  1. Ear. 2. Hearing. I. Title. [DNLM: 1. Ear—Anatomy and histology. 2. Ear—Physiology. 3. Hearing. WV272 H314a 1973]
  QP461.H3   612'.85   73-12474
  ISBN 0–672–61304–2

Anatomy and physiology of the peripheral hearing mechanism

Preface

This volume and its sequels, *The Electrophysiology and Layout of the Auditory Nervous System* and *Psychoacoustics,* are designed as texts for a one-semester course on the ear and hearing. Notes for this work were collected while teaching such a course in 1964 for ENT residents in otolaryngology at the University of Minnesota. I am grateful to Professor Frank Lassman for giving me this opportunity to teach. My gratitude also goes to Professor Moe Bergman for the opportunity progressively to update the notes to serve the needs of advanced students in this specialty at the Graduate Center of the City University of New York from 1966 to 1969; also to Professor Gene Powers for offering the same opportunity in connection with courses for Junior and Senior majors in the Department of Speech at the University of Connecticut, 1970–1973.

A recommended preliminary for the student using these volumes is a semester of experimental, or, preferably, physiological psychology, or a minimum of one semester of introductory speech pathology/audiology, which will familiarize him with anatomy, neurophysiology and psycho-

4 Anatomy and physiology of peripheral hearing mechanism

acoustics. The student may find some titles listed in the Suggested Readings at the back of this volume which will be helpful both for background reading and for further study.

J. D. H.

Introduction

In the human animal, the sense of hearing has developed to a near-miraculous degree the ability to detect and discriminate acoustic stimuli. Within the octaves of frequency to which we are most sensitive, no other animal surpasses us in picking up the faintest signal, while over very broad ranges of frequency and intensity, trained ears can recognize changes of one part of frequency in a thousand and variations of a quarter-decibel of intensity. They can distinguish to a few millionths of a second between the arrival time of the same stimulus at the two eardrums. These are very great biological achievements to which each detail of the auditory system, even the tiniest, makes its contribution, from the acoustically opaque pinna, or auricle, of the external ear to the frequency-specific layout of Stotler cells in the medial superior olivary nucleus in the brain stem.

The problems solved by Nature in developing and shaping our ears are difficult indeed: How to design a system which will respond to all frequencies, as does the ear of the moth, yet is sharply frequency-dependent and approaching critical damping; how to allow a dynamic range of intensity up to 1:1 billion, yet throughout this staggering range to accomplish almost equally good relative discrimination; how to quiet internal noise so that flapping of the eardrum, tremor of the stapedius muscle, coursing of blood around and through sensory cells, do not in fact deafen us to all but the loudest sounds; and how to arrange discrimination in microseconds when in fact the "grain" of the system—speeds of propagation of the nervous impulse, synapse latency—is a thousand times slower, of the order of milliseconds. In addition, all this must occur within a volume smaller than the end of one's little finger, with a truly tiny expenditure of energy, and buffered from all changes in the body posture and from the widest range of conditions of the body's food and gas intake or of ambient temperature, pressure, and humidity.

It is the aim of this work to review the capabilities of the human ear and to explore in some depth what is known about the anatomic-physiological substratum upon which these capabilities rest. Some notion will be given as to what can go wrong with the system or any of its parts, as well as how to ascertain in a quantitative fashion the nature of such dysfunction. We ask, for example, to what aspect of an acoustic stimulus we respond, whether to some feature of particle motion (displacement, acceleration, velocity) or of wave motion (pressure, acceleration, velocity). We seek to know the frequency range of the acoustic spectrum within which our ears respond, and the dynamic intensity range within which we operate. It is important to know the differences in aural sensitivity to simple and to progressively more complex signals, including speech. We must know how acuity is affected by duration of the stimulus, by repetition rate, and by the presence of other simultaneous stimuli. We may wish to examine how sensitivity data are affected by the subject's judgmental attitudes and tasks. In the case of binaural hearing, we seek to know whether and under what conditions the contralateral ear can affect an ear's response. We need to know what adaptations and fatigues the ear is susceptible of. And so on.

It seems impossible to consider these essentially psychoacoustic questions without exploring in some depth the anatomic-physiological bases on which these capabilities exist. The reader is invited therefore to follow some brief discussions as to how the acuities and sensitivities of the ear are provided for and shaped by the structures and arrangements of the auditory mechanism.

Arrangements of the auditory mechanism

The auditory mechanism may be viewed as being divided into three sections, the outer and middle ear and the spiral cochlea of the inner ear, each making its specific contribution to the hearing process. The outer ear is visible to us as an opaque appendage—the auricle or pinna—and a short tube—the external auditory (acoustic) meatus—leading to the middle ear cavity (tympanum) in the temporal bone.

Stretched across the opening between the outer and middle ear is the tympanic membrane, or eardrum, which communicates with a chain of three small bones, the ossicles (malleus, incus, and stapes), balanced delicately in, and occupying much of the air-filled tympanic cavity. A passageway, the Eustachian tube, leads from the tympanum to the nasopharynx and aids in maintaining the air pressure in the tympanum.

At the eardrum, the acoustic energy of the sound wave becomes mechanical energy and is passed on by action of the ossicles, through a small opening in the inner wall of the tympanum, the oval window (vestibular fenestra), to the fluid-filled vestibule of the inner ear. The footplate of the stapes, controlled by and held in place by the annular ligament, fits into the oval window as a stopper and, acting in response to movements of the other ossicles, presses in on, or pulls away from, the inner ear fluids, creating fluid motion (see plate one).

The labyrinth of fluid-filled spaces in the temporal bone includes the utricle, saccule, and the semi-circular canals (the so-called vestibular organ), which help maintain the body's equilibrium; and the cochlea. The latter is a spiral structure hollowed out of bone and coiled like a snail shell, which, unrolled, would measure about 1½ inches in length. Extending outward from the bony spine of the spiral (the modiolus), is a membranous canal, the scala media, stretching from the basal end of the cochlea almost to its apex. The scala media is filled with endolymph, a fluid continuous throughout the vestibular organ by way of the canalis reuniens. Above and surrounding this central sac is another canal, the scala vestibuli, and below it, the scala tympani, both filled with perilymph, another fluid, and connecting at the apex of the cochlea through a small hole, the helicotrema.

When the footplate of the stapes moves inward, the perilymph may flow up the scala vestibuli, around the tip of the scala media through the helicotrema, and down the scala tympani to this canal's termination in an

8 **Anatomy and physiology of peripheral hearing mechanism**

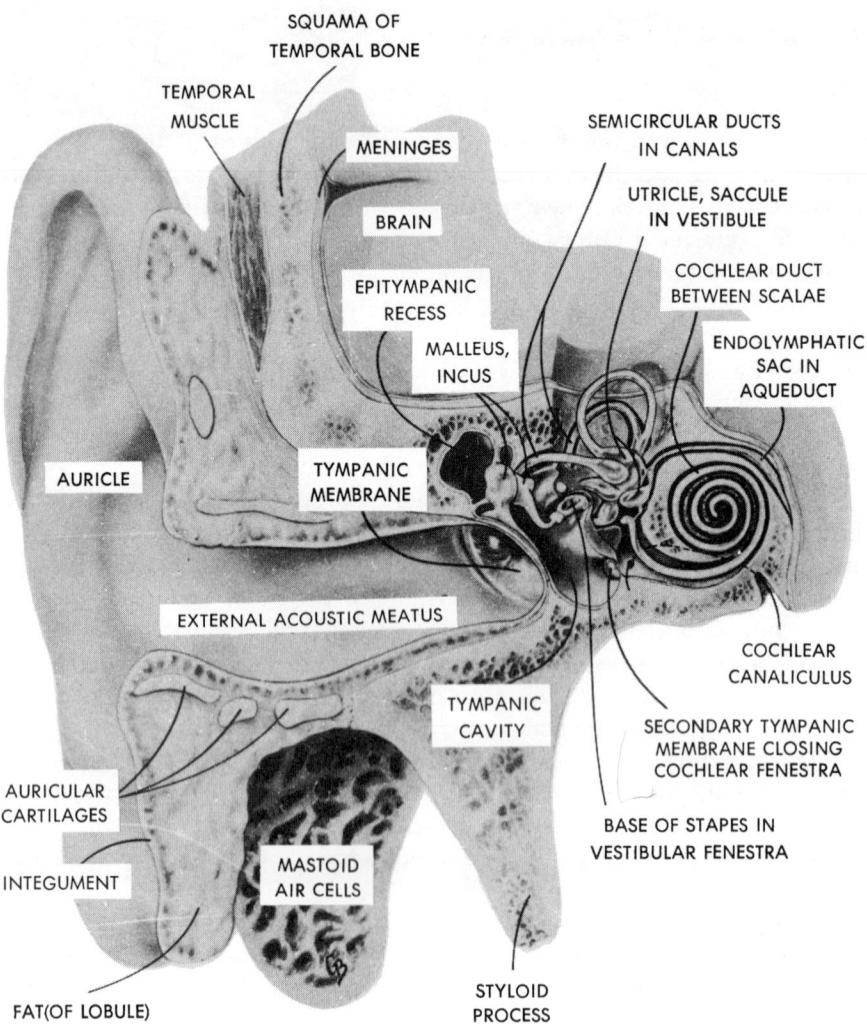

Plate I *The ear. (Anson and Donaldson 1967.)*

elastic membrane covering a second opening between the inner and middle ear, the round window, which serves as a pressure release.

The floor of the scala media is composed mainly of the flat basilar membrane, upon which is laid the organ of Corti, a complex structure containing the sensory or hair cells and their stereocilia (see figure 11, p. 40). The dendrites of the auditory nerve fibers originate close to the base of the hair cells. The ceiling of the scala media is a thin partition, Reissner's membrane.

When the ossicular chain is activated by acoustic pressure, the result is movement in the scala vestibuli and displacement of the scala media and its basilar membrane. A shearing action between the basilar membrane and the tectorial membrane which overlies the stereocilia somehow moves the stereocilia and stimulates the hair cells in the organ of Corti. They in turn excite the dendrites of the auditory nerve fibers. The impulse then travels from the auditory nerve to the auditory nuclei and tracts of the central nervous system, eventually reaching the cortex of the brain.

The acoustic stimulus

Imagine a ping-pong ball in a large echo-free field, contracting and expanding by some internal force 100 times per second. Spherical sound waves of alternate condensations and rarefactions of those air particles near the surface of the ball are created at the rate of 100 per second. Each particle of air affected moves back and forth along a radius of the ball at about the same distance (displacement) and velocity (speed) of the surface of the ball.

Now, particle motion results in wave motion, as each affected particle sets in motion other particles in expanding spherical waves, and we speak of a sound wave propagated outward from the ball. As the ping-pong ball creates rhythmic condensations and rarefactions of the medium, cyclic changes occur at every affected point in the air surrounding the ball. Thus a graph of the pressure changes over time at a point, say, 1 foot away from the ball, would show a slight sinusoidal variation of the normal ambient pressure. This pressure variation would be too small to be picked up by the usual barometer, but a pressure-sensitive microphone placed at that point and connected to an oscilloscope would in fact display the sinusoidal pressure variations. From these, the amplitude of particle displacement could be calculated according to a well-known formula.

A condensation (heightened pressure) at the outer side of the eardrum, combined with a constant pressure on the inner side, causes the eardrum to move inward, the extent of movement being governed by the pressure differential across the eardrum. Over wide frequency and intensity ranges, the movement of the eardrum is equal to, or of the same order of magnitude as, the displacement of air particles in the sound wave impinging on the eardrum. Conversely of course, a rarefaction in the external auditory meatus causes the eardrum to move outward.

Our ears give us no notion of the cyclic nature of the acoustic event; they act as might a meter attached to the pressure microphone—it does not register the moment-to-moment fluctuations of pressure as the oscilloscope does, but rather some running average of the pressure fluctuations over the duration of one or more cycles.

The acoustics of the head in a sound field

The baffle effect   When a plane progressive wave encounters an obstacle, a rearrangement of the sound field takes place. If a rigid sphere is inserted, for example, the sound pressure on the surface of the sphere closest to the sound source can be calculated or actually measured to be about 6 decibels (dB) greater than at the same point in space with the sphere removed (Wiener 1947). This 6 dB is for the case of a frequency of 1 kilocycle per second (kc/s) and a sphere about the size of the human head.

Of course, the human head is not a perfect sphere but appreciably flatter on the side aspect, the flat surface increasing the baffle effect somewhat. An actual measure of the baffle effect was taken by Wiener and Ross (1946). Figure 1 shows the case of the human head for angles of incidence of sound looking into the test ear, from straight ahead, and from 45°. Very appreciable diffraction effects are found up to 7 dB, exceeding 5 dB at most frequencies from 0.5 kc/s upward, when the sound source looks directly into the ear. It is for this reason that one turns the head not toward a faint sound if it is desired to apprehend it more clearly, but to a 90° angle of regard (azimuth).

The sound shadow effect   When a sphere is inserted into a sound field, the distribution of pressures around the sphere is dependent upon the azimuth from which the sound comes. For frequencies higher than about 1 kc/s, if the head is positioned so that the sound is directed toward one ear, the other ear may be in a sound shadow of some appreciable extent. The experimental technique is to move a sound source around the head, at a

11 Acoustics of the head in a sound field

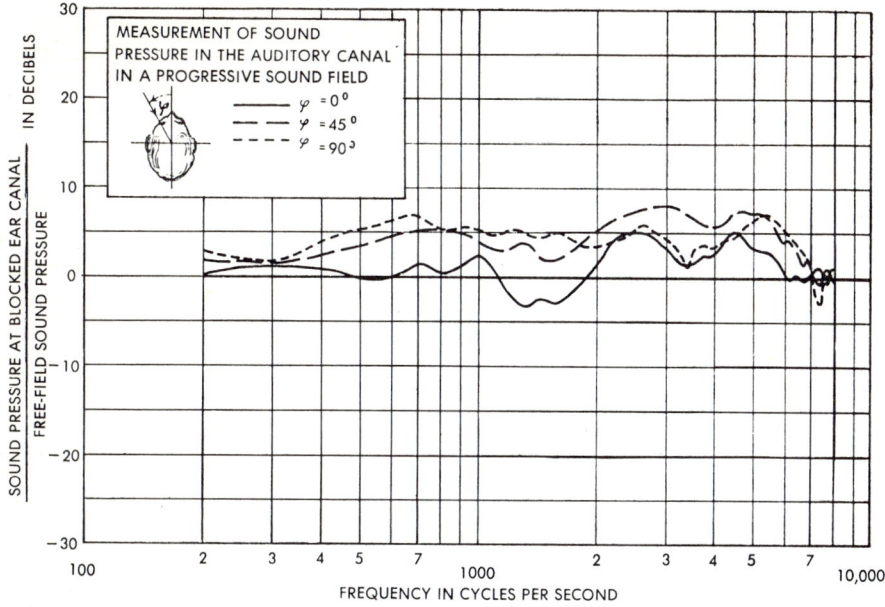

Figure 1 *The baffle effect. Ratio in decibels of the sound pressure at the blocked auditory canal to free-field sound pressure. (Wiener and Ross 1946.)*

succession of frequencies, measuring the sound pressure level (SPL) at the entrance to the (plugged) meatus, with either an actual head or an artificial head. Sivian and White (1933) outlined the main effects, and Wiener (1947) provided more complete treatment. The most careful and complete series of measurements on a really satisfactory artificial head, including realistic auricles or pinnae, were provided by Nordlund (1962), a selection of whose now classic results are in figure 2.

The contribution of the pinna A subsidiary question concerns the specific contribution of the pinna. It is clear, from our custom of cupping the ears with our hands, that some collecting if not amplification is accomplished by such structures. This must consist in some form of diffraction, since true reflection cannot occur from a surface whose area is small with respect to the wavelength of the incident sound. Also, of course, it has been suggested by experimentalists for over fifty years that the pinnae are important in front-back and in verticality localization of sounds.

12 Anatomy and physiology of peripheral hearing mechanism

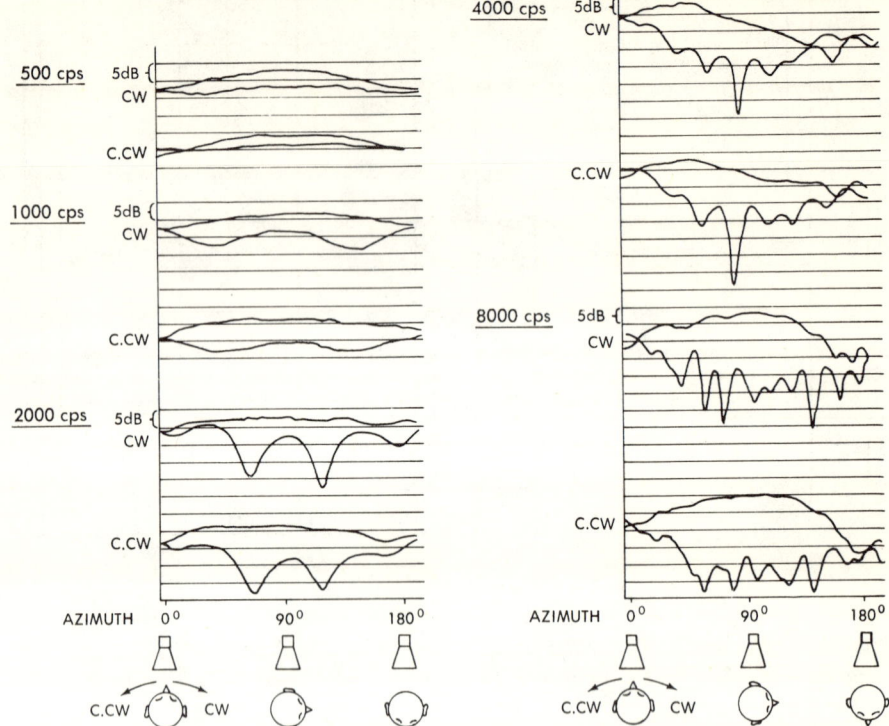

Figure 2 *The sound shadow. Registration of the intensity at the "eardrums" as a function of the azimuth of the sound source. (Nordlund 1962.)*

The human pinna is an acoustically opaque appendage, with surprisingly little variation among the world's peoples. Batteau (1967) has suggested that its surfaces provide temporal delay-lines to the eardrum, useful in monaural localization of sounds, particularly those overhead. His theory does not show clearly why the vertical dimension should be especially discriminable by time delays.

The writer has approached the problem (1972) using an artificial head with replaceable pinnae, one set perhaps overly large for the average, and the other set from a six-year-old boy (the writer is grateful to Todd Harris for permitting the plaster of Paris transfer technique eventuating in flexible replicas of the pinnae.) Sound shadows for specific frequencies can be drawn on polar plots so that a concentric circle can represent the condition

13 Acoustics of the head in a sound field

with no pinna at all, and deviations along radii from this circle can represent, frequency by frequency, the effect of the pinna itself, rather than of the whole head and pinna, as in figure 2. Sizable effects of the pinna are seen, but surprisingly enough, the effect of the pinna is not always, nor even usually, to increase, but actually to decrease, the interaural intensity difference.

It is to be emphasized, that the sound shadows thrown by a human head are not at all regular with frequency, azimuth, or elevation, so that interpolation between frequencies or azimuths or elevations is not justified even for the same head, while from head to head the differences may be very appreciable. The case seems to be that if one listens by way of earphones and probe-tube microphones to the acoustic conditions at another person's eardrums, some re-learning of our auditory world is necessary.

The canal resonance effect   Helmholtz tells us that when the length of a closed tube is ¼ the wavelength of a sound wave, a condition of resonance is set up, but that if the acoustic damping within the tube is relatively high, the tuning will not be very sharp. The case of the ear canal has been investigated by Wiener and Ross (1946) who compared the sound field at the entrance to the ear canal with that very close to the eardrum. A small-bore probe-tube extension to a microphone was pushed into the meatus by means of a fine-pitch screw, under otoscopic control. Angle from which the sound came was immaterial. Their data are shown in figure 3, reaching an effect of 10 dB at 3–4.5 kc/s. We see now that this must be so, since the average length of the meatus is about 2.5 cm, which is ¼ the wavelength of a tone of about 3.5 kc/s at body temperature. Thus the meatus is seen to have a broad resonance at a frequency region related to its length, tuned ± 2 octaves.

The influence of the whole head upon SPL at the eardrum   We are now ready to state the relation between the SPL (sound pressure level) at a point in space, before the head is introduced, and the SPL at the eardrum, with the head appropriately positioned. One combines the baffle effect, the head-shadow effect, and the canal-resonance effect. This has been done in figure 4. It is perhaps interesting to note that by using a baffle-and-tube construction Nature has not only protected the system but also created up to a 20-dB advantage, at the very critical 3–8 kc/s frequency region, over the solution of mounting the eardrum on the end of a tubular extension from the head, where neither a baffle nor a resonance could assist.

14 Anatomy and physiology of peripheral hearing mechanism

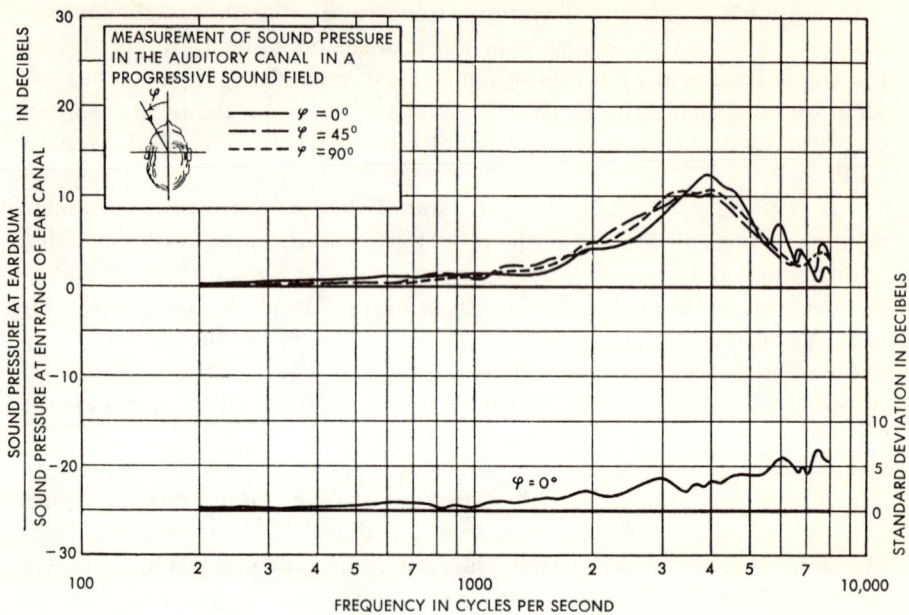

Figure 3 *The ear canal resonance effect. Ratio of the sound pressure at the eardrum to the sound pressure at the entrance to the auditory canal (average of 6–8 male ears). (Wiener and Ross 1946.)*

The eardrum

We now have both a general and a particular notion of the threshold SPL at the eardrum, and of the influence of body structure on the frequency spectra of the signals which reach the eardrum. One next asks, What of the eardrum? Does it set any limits to sensitivity, does it have frequency-dependent characteristics, etc.?

Anatomy The eardrum is almost transparent, very thin (0.07 mm) and elastic. In its resting state it is not, however, under much tension. Upon dissection it does not collapse but retains its shape as a little conical loudspeaker. It is set into the external meatus at a considerable slant (55°) from the perpendicular so that it is in fact not round but ellipsoid (axis

15 The eardrum

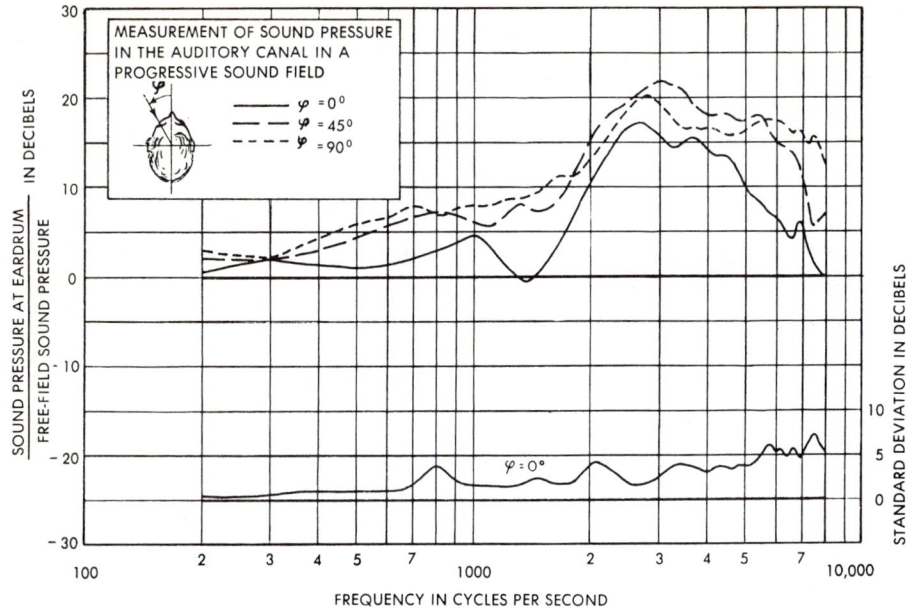

Figure 4 *Sum of the acoustic effects of the head. The ratio in decibels of the sound pressure at the eardrum to the sound pressure in the free field at the center of the listener's head (average of 6–12 male ears). (Wiener and Ross 1946.)*

ratio about 95:82), in order to increase its effective area without demanding of the meatus a larger bore. In the human, it has a total area of about 63.3 sq. mm. It does not, at the weaker SPLs, move in and out as a piston in a direction parallel to the meatus, but adopts a motion as a whole, hinged at the top. The axis of this rotation is in fact above the upper edge of the eardrum. The bottom section is capable of greater stretch to make this mode possible. Thus, faint sounds do not have to stretch large portions of the membrane unduly, but can simply rock it in the mode which offers least resistance, namely, by stretch movements in the lowest quadrant only. It is evident from these considerations that the mode of action of the eardrum at various intensities is very complex indeed.

The mass of the eardrum is reduced to the minimum by utilizing three layers only, an outer consisting of extremely thin skin, continuous with the lining of the meatus, but without cilia, or sebaceous (cerumen-forming)

16 Anatomy and physiology of peripheral hearing mechanism

and other specialized cells; a middle layer of radial and circular fibers, and an inner layer of gossamer mucous membrane which lines the whole middle ear even to the tiniest ligament.

Blood supply The inner and outer surfaces of the eardrum have different vascular sources, but for both, blood supply arises ultimately from the internal maxillary artery. There are many communications between the two sides, and manifold anastomoses, or joinings of blood vessels. If any vessel is cut, the anastomoses insure continuity of circulation. There is a noticeable plexus of vessels in the region of the manubrium (handle of the malleus) and another in a ring around the periphery of the eardrum. The indication is that the blood flow is from the manubrium outward, with the rich vein plexus collecting on the inner side and discharging mainly through veins in the middle ear.

Action The eardrum is markedly conical, pointing inwards (obtuse angle of about 150°); thus its sensitivity to high tones, or frequencies, is increased. A blunt termination of the ear canal would have given a pronounced bass boost, as does the skin of a bass drum. The eardrum's radial fibers, distributed rather evenly from the umbo at the center to the periphery, give it considerable undifferentiated stiffness, but its circular fibers are grouped into two concentric circles, one near the periphery and one much nearer the umbo, much as a good home hi-fi loudspeaker cone is crimped and rolled at the edges to increase the "flatness" of its frequency response.

In fact, the eardrum can best be thought of as a miniature loudspeaker cone, but in reverse: instead of accepting mechanical motion from electromagnetic force and transducing it into acoustic energy by moving the air, as a loudspeaker does, the eardrum responds to acoustic events over wide ranges of frequency and intensity, and transduces them into mechanical motion.

The manubrium of the malleus attaches to the eardrum at the upper boundary and extends to the center. The effect of this lengthened "point" of attachment seems to be to prevent loss of transmitted energy: if the malleus were attached to something approaching a true point at the center of the eardrum, a quantity of sound energy might be capable of moving some portion of the periphery of the eardrum, but not the critical portion at the center, with its added load of the ossicles.

17 **The eardrum**

Response to high intensities At moderately high intensities, the mode of vibration of the eardrum changes, operating less like a levered surface and more and more like a loudspeaker cone. A stroboscopically-illuminated motion picture by Kobrak (1959) of the rabbit eardrum exposed to more and more intense sound to the point at which the eardrum burst, shows at the highest intensities a flattened center section, with all the rest of the area clear to the peripheral attachment under severe stretch.

Acoustic events of an order of intensity which would be thought to rupture the eardrum are allowed for by providing general elasticity as well as stiffness. The eardrum is stiff enough to hold its circular and conical shape even when dissected free; nevertheless, large pressure changes in the meatus, whether alternating as in loud sounds or continuous as in altitude changes, are accommodated to a great extent by the ability of the whole surface of the eardrum to move inward. In the case of only moderately intense sounds, likewise, some of the modes of vibration over the surface of the eardrum reduce the excursion which the manubrium of the malleus would otherwise have to undergo. There is thus as a result of eardrum mechanics the first basis of a progressive nonlinearity between the intensity of the acoustic event and the actual movement of the ossicular chain.

Abnormal conditions The effect of partial destruction of the eardrum depends upon the type and area of defect. A small hole in the outer regions is without much effect, except at the lower frequencies. A large hole in the center is of course a different story. The integrity of the eardrum must be preserved enough to allow it to respond in phase with the acoustic event over at least a 30–40 dB range, and this energy transmitted to the manubrium, if usable hearing is to be in evidence. McArdle and Tonndorf (1968) have determined the effects of percentage of defect, and of quadrant, or location of defect, upon hearing in cat. Beginning at about 800 cycles per second (c/s), the influence of a perforation of only 5% increases as frequency is lowered, reaching about 30 dB at 250 c/s (i.e., at about −10 dB per octave), largely from the effect of admitting sound directly into the middle ear.

The eardrum itself is subject to infectious processes and distortions. The tissue may become infected and may finally perforate. A rupture can usually be seen with an otoscope, a small, illuminated, low-power magnifying instrument in common use. Also, the eardrum can become retracted

18 Anatomy and physiology of peripheral hearing mechanism

by absorption of air in the tympanum, when the tympanum is not aerated continually through the Eustachian tube. One is sometimes surprised by how far the eardrum is retracted—it may even be touching the cochlear promontory across the tympanum, and may be removed from there only by blowing air gently up the Eustachian tube (Politzerization).

A conclusion to be drawn is that the eardrum has a rather high safety factor. Although this membrane may be thickened, sustain small perforations, be drawn inward noticeably, or contain blebs within its layers, an audiogram, especially at high frequencies, may be relatively unaffected. The mistake is sometimes made of ascribing hearing defects to a "thickened eardrum" or "an old scar" when in fact the real trouble is more deeply rooted.

The ossicles and ossicular motion

Just as the eardrum is delicately and even beautifully modelled to collect a broad spectrum of acoustic energy, so the many interacting parts of the middle ear are equally well chiselled and combined (see plate 2). We have here a chain of three bones, each of complicated structure, each with relatively massy and relative fragile parts, with here and there facets and processes which seem to be without specific or overall plan. Yet, visualized suspended in the tympanum, with their numerous and strong attachments to the eardrum, to each other, to the annular ligament of the oval window, to the intratympanic muscles, and to the bony walls of the tympanic cavity, the ossicular chain is seen exquisitely made to rock around an imaginary fore-and-aft axis much as an inverted, V-shaped lever might rock around the point of the V, and to be very strongly restrained from rocking around any *other* axis, or indeed to move in any way at all except in this rocking. Thus the ossicular chain maintains its exact position in the tympanum, and attains its optimum rocking motion with almost unbelievably small movements of the eardrum, no matter what the position of the head in space (see figure 5).

The malleus and malleoincudal joint The manubrium of the malleus is tightly bound to the middle layer of the eardrum from just below the center of the membrane to the periphery at the top. Thus the center of

19 **Ossicles and ossicular motion**

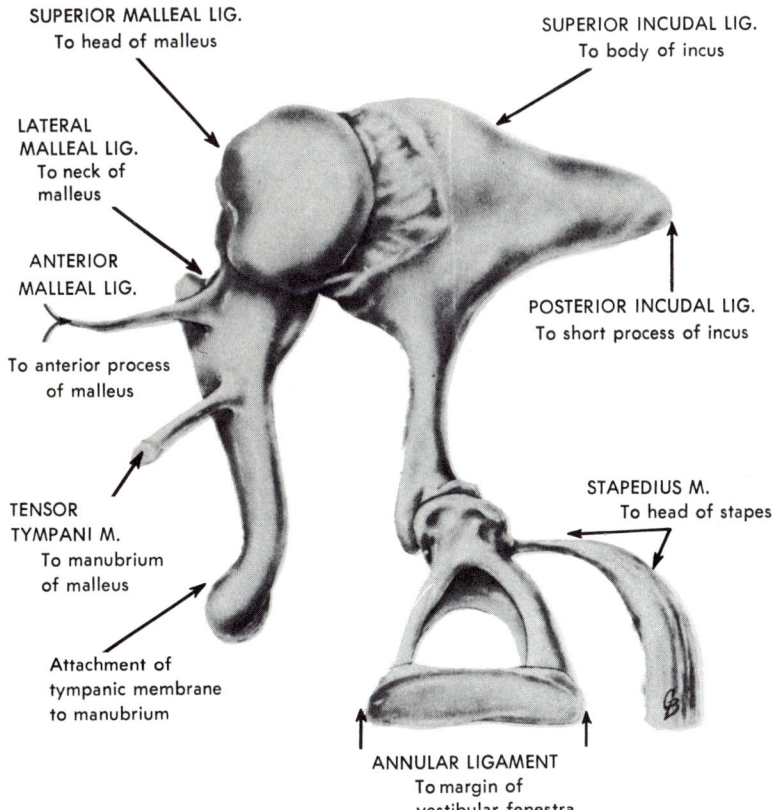

Plate II *The middle ear. (Anson and Donaldson 1967.)*

gravity of the capitulum (head of the malleus) is well above the upper rim of the eardrum. A short process of the malleus touches the eardrum near its upper margin and this projection seems to push the eardrum slightly outward, at the lower edge of a small inelastic triangle known as Schrapnell's membrane, or *pars flaccida*. This bony intrusion into the meatus can be seen clearly with the otoscope.

The ossicles depend upon vessels in the mucous membrane for blood

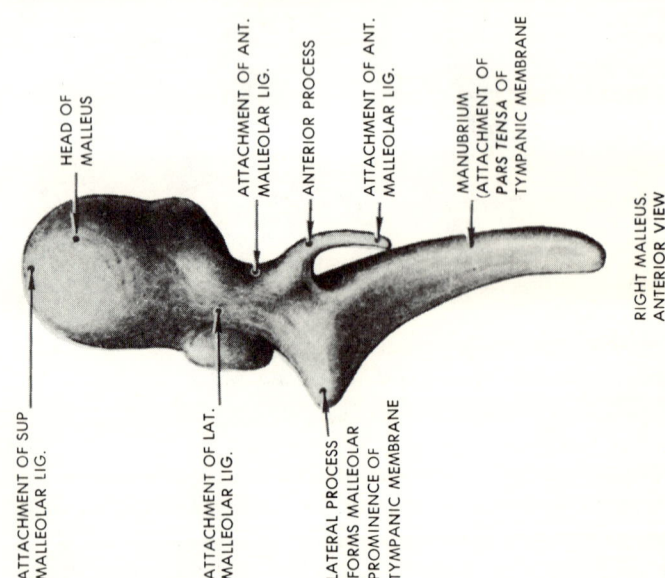

Figure 5 *The ossicles. (Truex and Kellner 1948.)*

21 Ossicles and ossicular motion

supply (figure 6). Two nutrient twigs from the superior branch of the anterior tympanic artery (see Anson, Harper, and Winch 1964) branch over the head of the malleus before the artery disappears into the bone. The interior of the manubrium is less well supplied. There is a capillary network in the mucous membrane covering the whole bone.

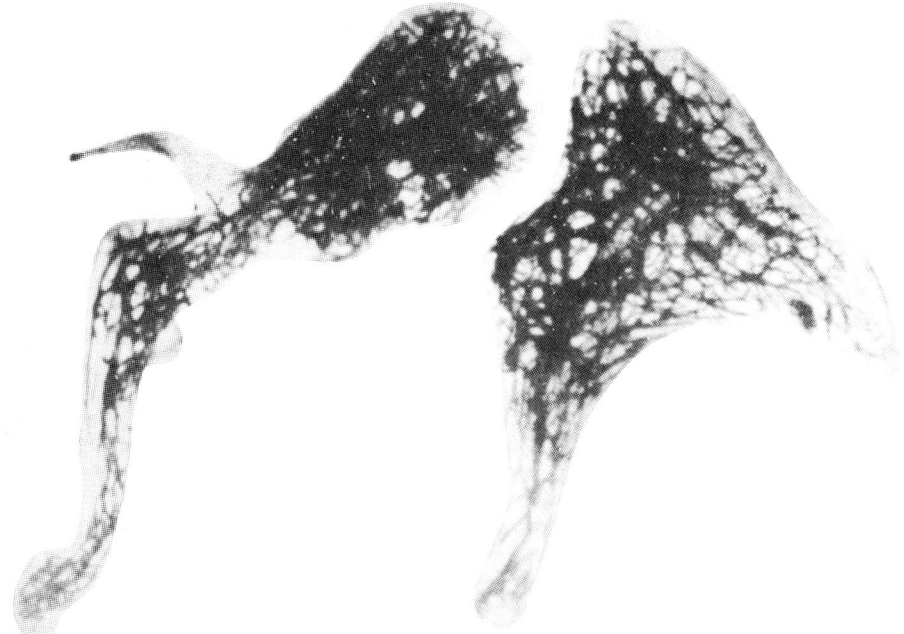

Figure 6 *Ossicular blood supply. (Kirikae 1960.)*

The 25-milligram (mg) mass of the malleus is connected to the walls of the tympanum from above, to the front, and to the back by three suspensory ligaments, and can be pulled inward by the ligament of the tensor tympani muscle (see plate II). Finally, the malleus is supported on the inward side by a relatively strong joint with the incus. This is a double-knuckle joint, each bone having a convex and a concave surface fitting each the other bone in reciprocity, so that if the arms of the joint are brought toward each other, the bones move in the bottom ball-and-socket; while if the arms are separated, they move on the upper ball-and-socket.

Thus the bones are never really disengaged. The joint is encapsulated so thoroughly that except for rather intense sounds the malleus and incus act as a single bone. The single bone of the bird's middle ear teaches us that this is also an efficient energy-transmission system, and that the joints between the ossicles in the vertebrate are there rather to reduce efficiency of sound transmission, as for dangerously intense pressure changes, than to render the ear more efficient at the usual pressure gradients encountered by the organism.

The incus and incudostapedial joint   The 25-mg mass of the incus, tightly bound as it is to the malleus, has two other supports. One of these is a tendon which attaches to its short process and goes straight back to the wall of the tympanum, approximately along the axis of rotation of the malleus-incus mass. The other is its attachment to the stapes, a relatively fragile joint. Its long, or lenticular process, which forms the downward-going arm of the V lever, bends inward at the bottom before attaching to the head of the stapes. This incudostapedial joint, while encapsulated, is nevertheless easily disjointed by sudden outward movement of the incus, as with sudden reduction of pressure in the meatus.

Theoretically, the axis of rotation of the malleus-incus unit would be most efficient if placed so that it passed through the center of gravity of their combined mass (including the not quite negligible mass of the eardrum and stapes); and this has been established by Kirikae (1960) (see figure 7). He found the center of gravity by hanging the ossicles from a spider thread in several attitudes and determined the axis of rotation to pass through the center and the axis to lie in the expected plane just above the eardrum. Thus the eardrum must pivot not exactly on its upper edge, but on an imaginary axis just above this line.

Two small blood vessels from the superior branch of the anterior tympanic artery penetrate the body and long process of the incus, and one from the posterior branch of the anterior tympanic artery goes to the posterior process. All three make up an extremely rich network in the mucosa covering the incus. In the long process especially, the intra-bone circulation is poor (see Hamberger and Wersäll 1964), the bone depending heavily on the mucosa. If the mucosa is eroded or strangulates, the lenticular process would be endangered; and indeed this process is often seen damaged in patients with middle ear pathology.

The stapes   The 2.5-mg mass of the stapes is so tiny that it is supported

23 Ossicles and ossicular motion

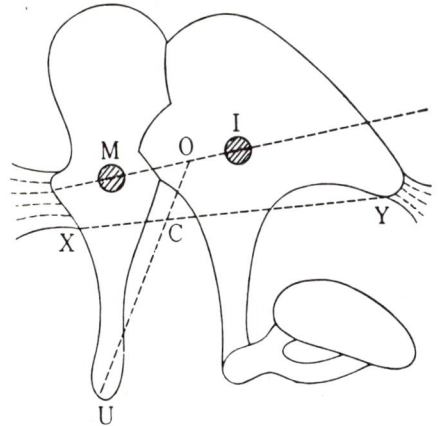

Figure 7 *Ossicular axis of rotation. M: center of gravity of malleus; O: center of gravity of malleus-incus block; I: center of gravity of incus; U: tip of mallear handle; C: center of gravity of conductive system; X–Y: rotation axis of ossicular chain. (Kirikae 1960.)*

quite sufficiently by the annular ligament investing the edge of the footplate (see plate 2). The tendon which attaches to the stapedius muscle and inserts on the caput, or head, of the stapes has no supporting function.

The stapes is supplied with blood mainly from a branch of the stylomastoid artery. There may be no vessels at all in the bone of the crura, or cross sections, and few in the footplate, so that these portions are dependent upon mucosal circulation.

The engineering construction of the stapes, with its great strength per unit mass, is a biological triumph. Its main cross sections, from head to footplate, are hollow, each extremely thin crus shaped in the form of a gothic arch, one of the strongest arches possible. Inasmuch as the transmission of higher frequencies of vibration through any mechanically vibrating system is better when the mass of the system is slight, the carving away of the mass of the stapes must profoundly increase the range of high frequencies to which the ear is sensitive.

Note that it is more important for the stapes to be light than for the malleus-incus: the latter mass is balanced around the axis of rotation, so that the lightest touch on its first level arm, at the umbo, would start it vibrating, even were its mass doubled or tripled; but the stapes is a dead weight on the incus that would take twice the energy to drag back and forth if its weight were double. It seems now so light as almost to crumple when called upon to push so strongly, as it must push against the fluid at the oval window. If it were not for its arch-like construction, it would indeed crumple.

The footplate of the human stapes does not in fact move in and out of the oval window exactly as a piston (though it may do so in the cat). The movement of the lenticular process of the incus is not exactly in line with the position of the stapes, but a trifle forward. Thus the footplate rather pivots on a vertical axis passing through its posterior, much as a door moves on its hinges. The thickness of the footplate tapers somewhat to accommodate this type of strain, and the annular ligament has about three times the depth of the accordion pleat at its front than at its back portion, to accommodate the greater anterior excursion.

According to Békésy (1960), at acoustic intensities of 70 dB SPL and higher in the meatus, the footplate begins to take on, largely as the result of stapedial activity, a new mode of vibration. Finally, at very high intensities, its axis is turned horizontal, as a door might rotate over a horizontal rod fixed in the middle from the left jamb to the right jamb, so that as the top swings in, the bottom swings out, and vice versa. As a consequence, a short circuit is created: as the acoustic intensity in the meatus increases, the footplate no longer operates like a piston to drive larger and larger volumes of fluid through the inner ear. Instead, the footplate motion allows for fluid pushed in at the top of the door to be compensated for by fluid pushing out at the bottom of the door. Thus, fluids further into the cochlear ducts are not in motion because the pressure is equalized through a shunt. So far as the inner ear is concerned, then, high pressures in the meatus never have their full effect on the delicate structures resting on the basilar membrane.

Gross anatomy and innervation of the intratympanic muscles

Tensor tympani This muscle is about 25 mm long, in cross section about 5 sq mm, lying for the most part within a bony canal parallel to the Eustachian tube. Its ligament goes upward to the level of the umbo, then around a small spicule of bone and thence across the tympanum to its attachment on the manubrium of the malleus, somewhat above the umbo (see plate 2). Its histology is unique (see Gerhardt, David, and Marx 1966). Its muscle fibers are striate and unstriate, short and parallel, interspersed liberally with fatty tissue, indicating a very active muscle. Presumably it is the striate fibers which in some persons are under voluntary control. In the rabbit, the resting tendon exerts a pull of 0.5 grams (g) and it is likely that this is approximately correct for the human.

25 Gross anatomy and innervation of intratympanic muscles

The innervation of the muscle is quite complex. The main supply is the mandibular branch of cranial nerve V through the otic ganglion, a mass of nerve cells and tissues also serving the orbital region, but it is believed that other supply exists:

1) A branch of cranial nerve IX goes to the inner wall of the middle ear and breaks up into the tympanic plexus (see figure 8). One fascicle of

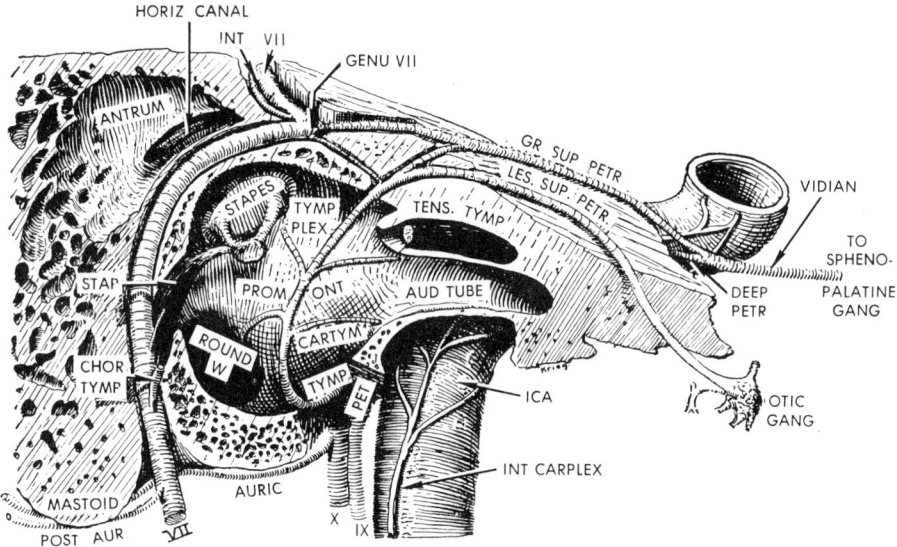

Figure 8 *The tympanic plexus. Tymp. plex.: tympanic plexus; promont.: promontory of cochlear capsule; aud. tube: Eustachian tube; gr. sup. ptr.: greater superficial petrosal nerve; les. sup. ptr.: lesser superficial petrosal nerve; tens. tymp.: tensor tympani muscle; chor. tymp.: chorda tympani (cranial nerve VII) (Krieg 1953.)*

this plexus travels near the tensor tympani, giving off fibers to the insertion end of the muscle, then leaves the cranial cavity as the lesser superficial petrosal nerve, and ends in the otic ganglion. Whether these twigs to the tensor tympani are motor or sensory, Lawrence (1962) could not determine. They seemed not to be sympathetic fibers to the vascular system in the muscle.

2) Kobrak (1959) states that there are parasympathetic afferent fibers from the geniculate ganglion of cranial nerve VII, which presumably reach the smooth muscle fibers.

3) There is the possibility that some of the fibers from the otic ganglion are post-ganglionic fibers from the sympathetic chain.

Stapedius This muscle in the human is about 6–7 mm long, in cross section about 5 sq mm, lying vertically in a bony canal in the pyramidal eminence, a blunt projection of the cochlear capsule, posterior to the stapes. Its tendon emerges from a tiny canal in the pyramidal eminence and bends sharply in the horizontal plane to attach to the neck of the stapes and the incudostapedial joint. It is characterized by an unusually rich neural supply, small motor unit size, and limited sensory innervation. The adult human stapedial nerve (an offshoot of cranial nerve VII) enters the muscle and immediately splits into three branches which go to different regions and arborize into a total of about 120 twigs, each one innervating 6 to 8 muscle fibers. In the newborn, each twig innervates about 21 muscle fibers, thus the reduction to 6–8 for the motor unit in the adult is seen to be in the direction of better control of delicate neuromuscular coordination.

A somewhat less rich sensory innervation is present; there are muscle spindles, and sensory endings within the tendon.

The site at which the parasympathetic fibers arise which supply the stapedius has not been definitely determined. It is presumed they come from the geniculate ganglion.

Action of the intratympanic muscles

Stimuli leading to tympanic muscle activity

1. *Direct observation of response to stimuli* Otologists for a century have noted that a muscle twitch can be seen in response to a sound led to either ear (see Lüscher 1929). In most patients with a perforated eardrum, movements of the tendons are easily visualized with only low-power optical magnification. Lindsay, Kobrak, and Perlman (1936), through a perforated eardrum, saw movement to a sound at 65–90 dB over the contralateral ear threshold for all frequencies the patient could hear. Kobrak (1959) succeeded in rendering the posterior superior quadrant of some normal eardrums almost transparent by chemical applications, and determined that contralateral pure tones about 60 dB above threshold were adequate stimuli for observable movement of the stapedius tendon.

The excursion of the stapes by action of the stapedius muscle is 0.2 mm (Kobrak 1948) for posterior movement of the capitulum (head) of the stapes, and 0.16 mm for outward movement of the anterior lip of the footplate. These movements are quite sufficient to partially disarticulate the incudostapedial joint.

Observations of patients with tetanized contractions of the tensor tympani reveal that when the muscle is relaxed by anesthesia, or its tendon cut, the eardrum, previously drawn strongly inward by the contractions, resumes its normal position. This can be observed with the otoscope.

2. *Measurement of stimuli through electrical output of muscles* The electrical output of the muscles in response to contralateral acoustic stimuli was first observed by Perlman and Case (1939), and since by Salomon and Starr (1963) and Djupesland (1965), among others. Subjects were usually patients with middle ears exposed on the operating table. Latency of activity in the stapedius is agreed upon as being only about 10 milliseconds (msec), pointing to only a very few synaptic relays even in the crossed stapedius reflex. Fisch and von Schulthess (1963) found that the electromyogram threshold for noise was about 70 dB SPL. Latency in the tensor tympani has been estimated variously as 80–280, and 90–300 msec, i.e., much longer than for the stapedius.

3. *Change in impedance as measure of stimuli* Many researchers since Metz (1946) have explored, by way of an impedance bridge, the stimuli leading to intratympanic muscle activity. Such a device determines the reduction in sound transmission through the middle ear as a result of any change in mechanical efficiency. Terkildsen (1960), for example, found the acoustic threshold of impedance change due to stapedius activity to be 75 dB SL (sensation level, or decibels above threshold) at 1 kc/s, with a latency of 57 ± 26 msec at 90 dB SL, and of 44 ± 11 msec at 110 dB SL. Deutsch (1968) recorded the acoustic output of the impedance bridge and found impedance changes at mean threshold of 62 dB SL for white noise, 62 dB SL for noise bands ⅓ octave in width centered at 2 or 4 k/s, and 73, 82, and 81 dB SL for pure tones of 0.25, 2, and 4 kc/s respectively.

The dynamic characteristics of stapedius action were studied by Dallos (1964), who continuously recorded the acoustic output of the impedance bridge. Transmission loss was almost linear with increasing SPL from threshold for the reflex (70–85 dB SPL) up to 110 dB, a range of 20–40 dB. At 110 dB it took 80–100 msec for the transmission loss to approach 80% of its maximum final value, and 700–1300 msec to drop 80% when the noise terminated. At threshold, the reflex effect adapted at the rate of

0.3 dB per sec, but at 105 dB and higher there was no adaptation at all.

The acoustic threshold for stapedius activity to pure tones was studied by Møller (1962). His figure 1 shows the threshold in dB SPL; not much muscle activity is generated by stimuli higher than 15 kc/s, and the lower frequencies fall off in much the same fashion as the threshold of hearing itself.

The situation is quite different in the tensor tympani. Klockhoff (1961) found no impedance changes at all to sound stimuli to 120 dB SL with 20 patients suffering from actual or functional loss of the stapedius reflex, but with mobile eardrum and incus, and presumably normal tensor tympani muscles. He thus concludes, with such earlier writers as Békésy and Lüscher, that no acoustic stimulus short of startle intensity will induce tensor tympani activity. He also showed that electric shock in the homolateral meatus (not the contralateral) elicited no impedance changes, though such a stimulus in normal ears is adequate to initiate stapedius activity. Evidently weak electric shock is an adequate stimulus for the homolateral stapedius but not for the tensor tympani.

Djupesland (1962) found that cutaneous stimulation of the meatus (or eardrum if the pinna and meatus were anesthetized) would initiate bilateral stapedius-like impedance changes. In unilateral deafness a cutaneous stimulus on the deaf side gave the usual reflex on the normal side, thus ruling out an afferent path of nerve VIII. He later confirmed (1964) that these cutaneous stimuli were consensual, but that electric shock was only homolateral.

When he attached a mechano-electric transducer to the tendons of 114 patients being operated on for stapes fixation, Djupesland found that the tensor tympani reflex was never elicited by meatal stimulation, but that it was easily elicited by voluntary or reflex contractions of the periorbital muscles. The best way to stimulate the tensor tympani without startle and without affecting the stapedius, was said to be to lift the upper eyelid manually.

Klockhoff and Anderson (1960) showed that a very brief change in impedance does occur, in patients with no stapedius reflex functional, when a puff of air is sent against the eye region. A rather wide trigeminal nerve area is capable of initiating such an afferent discharge. This can only be a brief, easily adapting twitch of the tensor tympani as part of a startle to a cutaneous rather than an acoustic stimulus. Such a reflex can have certain advantages as a diagnostic help in the clinic.

Klockhoff (1961) corroborated these results, and added that in six normal ears, in which the stapedius was already active in the response to sound, the orbital air jet added an increment to the response, with a latency of 60–90 msec. This is surely by way of tensor tympani activity, by reason of its long latency, its brief duration (0.5 sec), and its quick habituation.

The impedance method thus contributes the information that the stapedius is thrown into non-habituating bilateral activity very quickly to only moderately loud sounds, and also by cutaneous stimulation to either meatus, or electric shock to the homolateral meatus; and that the tensor tympani undergoes brief, quickly adapting twitches to sounds loud enough to startle, and to an unexpected stimulation of the orbital region.

4. *Rise in audiometric threshold*   This index cannot well be used with an acoustic stimulus, but Pichler and Bornschein (1957) showed that weak electric shock to the homolateral meatus can degrade (raise) the human threshold, presumably from stapedius activity.

Action of the muscles on the eardrum   Registration of changes in static air pressure within the external meatus, presumably reflects movements of the eardrum due to muscle activity. A first guess as to the possible action of the muscles separately on the eardrum would be that the tensor tympani pulls the eardrum inward, while the stapedius pushes it somewhat outward. Weiss et al. (1962) make this assumption in interpreting their data. Yet they show examples of some ears with a predominantly outward movement of the eardrum to sound of any level, others with a predominantly inward movement to the same stimuli. In others, an initial positive or negative pressure can change to a biphasic response.

Neergaard and Rasmussen (1966) point out that under some resting conditions of the eardrum, a displacement inward of the center of the eardrum could lead to either an inward or outward direction of the total volume displacement. When they introduced a -5 cm H_2O pressure in the meatus, their subjects gave first an inward movement, then a biphasic movement; when they introduced a $+5$ cm H_2O pressure, first an outward movement resulted, then a biphasic. Their results concerned only the stapedius muscle, inasmuch as the modal latency of the reflex recorded was only 15–17 msec, ruling out the later action of the tympani.

The results of Holst, Ingelstedt, and Örtegren (1963) bear on this matter. In 14 of 16 subjects, the tensor tympani reflex, upon the blowing of air into the eye region, gave an inward movement of the eardrum, as would be expected on mechanical grounds. However, 5 subjects gave

30 Anatomy and physiology of peripheral hearing mechanism

biphasic responses. An air jet into the contralateral meatus, known to elicit the stapedius reflex, gave outward movements in 11 of 16 subjects, the other 5 giving biphasic responses. Finally, with tones of 0.5 kc/s at 127 dB SPL, 13 of 16 subjects gave outward movements, 4 gave biphasic. With tones of this sort, both muscles would normally have contracted. In some of these subjects given a rapidly repeated series of tone bursts, the inward component of the biphasic response quickly adapted, leaving only the outward component. It seems clear here that the tensor tympani, known to adapt very quickly, was contributing to the inward component, the stapedius to the outward. However, it is also clear that the interpretation of any single record in these experiments is quite complex and correspondingly uncertain.

Action of the muscles in producing transmission loss The maximum action of the muscles in attenuating (reducing) sound was investigated by Neergaard et al. (1963). They applied tones to the eardrums of cadavers and recorded SPLs from a probe microphone sealed over the round window. The muscles were removed from their points of origin on the temporal bone, gauges were attached, and known forces applied, in excess of normal, through the tendons of the muscles. Losses in sound transmission may be seen in their figure 3 for each muscle separately. When tension was applied to both muscles simultaneously, the effect was strictly additive—both muscles work quite independently through any range of force encountered in nature. A pull on the stapedius increased the phase of the transmitted sound, compared with that of resting tension, as if from increased *stiffness* of the system, but a pull on the tensor tympani changed the phase little if at all, seemingly indicating increased friction.

The action of the stapedius in degrading human threshold was found by Pichler and Bornschein (1957) to be about 10–12 dB at 127–750 c/s, diminishing to zero at about 1.5 kc/s. These authors used electric shock to the homolateral meatus. Klockhoff and Anderson (1959) found with this same stimulus that the reflex adapts so quickly that audiometry should be unaffected; but Pichler and Bornschein's data were to some extent substantiated by Borg (1968), who found 12–14 dB attenuation to sound in response to a tone of 0.5 kc/s at 20 dB over reflex threshold, but attenuation of only 0–6 dB for a tone of 1450 c/s in patients with inactive tensor tympani muscles due to palsy of cranial nerve V.

The effects of muscle contraction on the audiometric threshold (see Reger et al. 1963, and Sherrick and Mangabeira-Albernaz 1961) and on suprathreshold loudness phenomena (see Loeb and Riopelle 1960; Loeb and Fletcher 1961; and Prather 1961) are still controversial (for review see Loeb 1964).

Liden, Nordlund, and Hawkins (1963) showed that speech discrimination in noise was relatively better in stapedectomy patients with the stapedius tendon preserved. They felt the stapedius might reduce masking of speech by attenuating low-frequency masking sounds and thus improve the speech/noise ratio.

The middle ear as a transducer of energy

It is often said that the function of the eardrum and middle ear is to "match" as closely as possible the acoustic impedance of the air in the meatus and the much greater impedance of fluids in the cochlea. Generally speaking, the acoustic impedance of a transmitting medium is the ratio of sound pressure exerted on the surface to the sound energy flux generated by that pressure through the medium. When an acoustic wave in any medium, such as air, comes to an interface with another medium, such as water, only some of the acoustic energy is absorbed by the second medium; the rest of the energy "bounces" back through the first medium as a reflected sound wave. The amount of acoustic energy absorbed by the second medium is greater, the closer the match of acoustic impedances.

If the eardrum and ossicles did not exist, and acoustic waves in the air impinged directly upon the oval window, 99.9% of the sound would be rejected at the interface and be reflected back into the air. This would be an inefficiency of about 30 dB.

The extremely efficient solution adopted by the mammalian middle ear is to accept nearly all the energy in the air but to transduce this acoustic energy into mechanical energy, namely, in-and-out movements of the whole eardrum-ossicular system. The extent of these eardrum-ossicle movements is about that of the movements of individual particles of air at the eardrum which drive the middle-ear structures. But note that these in-and-out movements of the eardrum-ossicle system are not expressions of acoustic energy, but mechanical energy. For acoustic energy to pass through the middle ear system, it would be necessary for waves of condensation-rarefaction to pass from eardrum to footplate, with successive physical points generally not in phase; but as in all mechanical systems the eardrum-ossicle system moves in and out as a unit, in phase at all points (though there is some phase lag at the highest frequencies).

Of course, about 0.1% of the acoustic energy in the ear canal is in fact transmitted as a series of condensations-rarefactions through the ossicles, but this energy is vanishingly small and can be completely ignored. Thus we are not at all concerned with acoustic energy in the middle ear. Rather, the problem of the mammalian middle-ear construction is how to transduce the acoustic waves of condensation-rarefaction of air, impinging on the eardrum, into mechanical vibratory movements of the ossicles.

Pressure amplification of the middle ear Wever and Lawrence (1954) presented evidence and arguments against Helmholtz's notion of the eardrum itself as a catenary lever (but see Tonndorf and Khanna, 1970). There remain as possibilities for pressure amplification (1) a mechanical leverage of the ossicles, and (2) a pressure amplification by way of the footplate being much smaller than the effective area of the eardrum.

Dahmann (1929) found the ossicular chain lever-arm ratio in the cadaver to be a reduction in movement of 1:1.31 from malleus to incus, giving a pressure amplification of 1.31. The ratio of the eardrum-footplate areas will differ widely from individual to individual. Wever and Lawrence (1954) give an average value of 64.3 sq mm for the total area of the eardrum, of which about ⅔, or 42.9 sq mm was said to be the effective area. The footplate measures 3.2 sq mm, which is all effective area; thus the pressure increase is $42.9/3.2 = 13.4$.

The lever effect can now be multiplied with the areal ratio, or $1.31 \times 13.4 = 17.5$, or 24.9 dB, which is one estimate of the pressure-transformation ratio in the human ear.

This figure of 25 dB is in very good agreement with measurements on the cadaver. Békésy in 1941 (see Békésy 1960) dissected and drilled a human temporal bone so that acoustic energy could be applied simultaneously at the eardrum and the stapes footplate. The sound pressure level (SPL) needed at the stapes to produce a null of stapes movement was measured. Phase and intensity adjustments were of course possible at the stapes, and the null in movement was measurable with a capacitance probe. The pressure transformation ratio was found to be about 24 dB gain at 2 kc/s as seen in his figure 5–4. Notice that it is almost independent of frequency up to 2400 c/s. Of course, in this experiment the stapes was not loaded by fluids as in the normal case, but then, neither was it moving. Onchi (1961) in a similar study gave data for an average of seven normal ears (see figure 9).

33 The middle ear as a transducer of energy

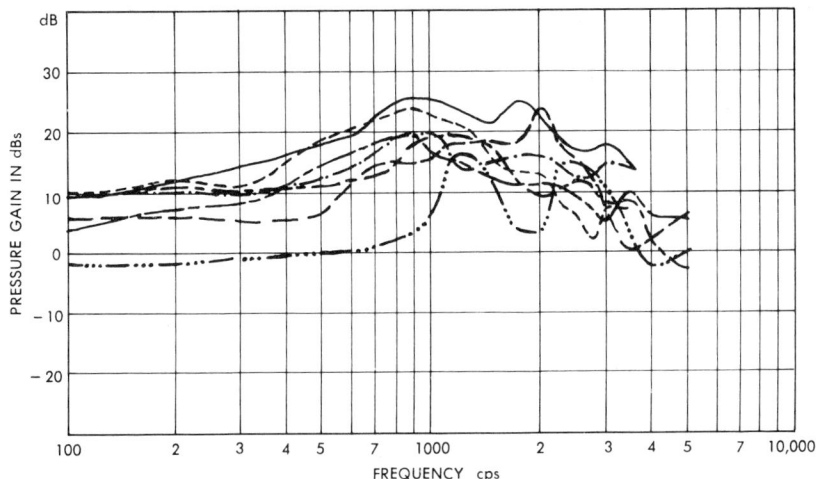

Figure 9 *Acoustic transmission through the middle ear. Apparent pressure gain recorded for seven ears. The thick curve is for a somewhat pathological ear. (Onchi 1961.)*

Now an amplification of 25 dB does not of course equal the 30-dB impedance mismatch of air and water as mentioned above. In cat, where this problem has been studied especially by Wever and Lawrence (1954), the entire 30-dB inefficiency is made up by the middle ear. Does the human do less well? Probably it does as well.

When one takes into consideration 1) that the actual pressure measurements in the cadaver present some problems of probe-tube calibration; 2) the low-tone sound leaks in Onchi's experiment; 3) the drying of the specimen, etc., which could easily cumulate to a slight loss; and 4) that the calculation of 24.9 dB rests on estimates of lever-arm length and effective areas which could well contain a $\pm$ 10% uncertainty (in this case $\pm$ 4.25 dB), it seems likely, from these uncertainties of experiment, and from what we know of the audiogram shifts of those patients with loss of all middle-ear structures, that the true transformation action of the human middle ear actually equals, or very nearly equals, the 30-dB impedance mismatch which the middle ear was designed to overcome.

In persons with no middle-ear structures except for the stapes footplate a loss of 45–60 dB exists, larger at the higher frequencies. This figure is contaminated by direct action of sound on the round window and is rather inexact since pre-operative audiograms accurate to within $\pm$ 5 dB, taken on these ears when absolutely normal are almost never available.

Frequency dependency in the middle ear The ossicular chain and supporting structures in the middle ear, as in every mechanical system, have their own period of vibration. If the lever arm at the umbo is tapped only once, it must tend to vibrate at its own natural frequency (depending on its mass and stiffness). The natural period of the middle-ear structures is about 1.5 kc/s, and if these are unloaded by the inner ear they would vibrate at that frequency for a time after the driving force is withdrawn. Of course, the stapes is heavily loaded by the cochlear fluids, which tend to damp the vibrations within a cycle or two.

The effect of the air-filled cavity in the middle ear must be considered. This cavity is shaped like a pocket watch, about 15 mm in radius, about 4–6 mm thick at the periphery, but only about 2 mm thick at the center. It has a volume of about 2 cc, of which one fourth to one third is taken up by the ossicles. It can be appreciated that such a small air bubble can present a considerable stiffness to movements inward of the eardrum, and can reduce low-frequency sensitivity by as much as 10 dB. In some animals, such as the desert rat, an increase in size of the middle-ear cavity has seemingly led to an exceptionally keen low-frequency hearing. (However, it must be considered that in this species, the eardrum/oval window areal ratio is also greatly increased.) Concomitantly, the larger cavity raises the resonant frequency so that the ear operates well over a wider high-frequency range.

Békésy in 1942 (see Békésy 1960) determined that the volume displacement of the round window was the same for all frequencies up to 1200 c/s for the same SPL in the external meatus. Since round window displacement must be very closely proportioned to stapes displacement, he concluded that the middle ear does not contribute to the low-frequency audiogram.

Wever (1949) fully treated the problem of the frequency-response characteristic of the audiogram, and concluded that the middle ear does not contribute much. The relation of frequency to sensitivity was predicted from the summation of six factors, only one of them being acoustic resonance.

Anderson, Hansen, and Neergaard (1964) repeated Békésy's data on round window volume displacement as a function of SPL. These authors reversed the direction of sound transmission by putting sound in at the round window and measuring SPL in the external meatus. This procedure increased efficiency by greatly reducing the amount of input SPL needed to yield usable (and, especially, distortion-free) results (see figure 10).

35 The middle ear as a transducer of energy

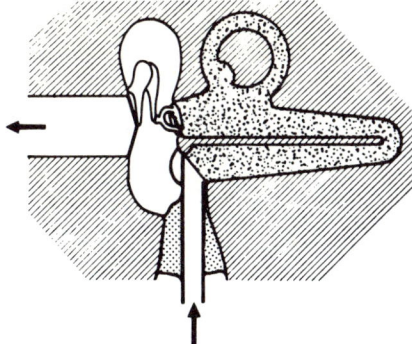

Figure 10 *Experimental study of acoustic transmission through the middle ear. (Anderson, Hansen, and Neergaard 1964.)*

The middle ear of the cadaver seems to be distortion free at least up to 110 dB SPL, where phase velocity is reduced from increased mass for frequencies over 500 c/s.

Rubinstein et al. (1966) studied stapes displacement for constant eardrum SPL with a capacitative probe in the human cadaver. The stapes was unloaded by the cochlea so that it may seem that the middle ear was being studied under perfectly isolated conditions. But the ossicular chain will certainly operate in a different fashion with the cochlea dissected away, and the data of Rubenstein et al. in their figure 6 can only approximate the actual conditions; their data show some roll-off for the lower frequencies, about 5–6 dB from 1 down to 0.1 kc/s.

Investigations generally agree that stapes displacement at unit SPL is constant for all frequencies at and below the natural period of the middle ear. At higher frequencies, the stapes amplitude falls off at the rate of about 12 dB/octave (i.e., with the square of frequency), and the phase of the stapes motion begins to lag behind the acoustic phase at the eardrum.

For a constant SPL at the eardrum, the volume of fluid displaced by the stapes is estimated by Guinan and Peake (1967) from their own and thirteen previous investigations, employing a variety of species and methods, to be from 0.02 to 4×10^{-6} cubic mm/dyne. The range in these estimations is a factor of 200 from least to most (200 x), and tells us that we do not have a final figure on the transmission efficiency of the mammalian ear. There is a range of 20 x even within those investigations all using the human cadaver. Møller's (1965) studies on middle ear impedance before and after severing the incudostapedial joint show that resistance (friction) is sharply reduced, but that stiffness and mass are little changed. Thus the loading of the inner ear is the major component; there is negligible energy loss, and little acoustic damping, in the middle ear itself.

When Guinan and Peake (1967) computed stapes displacement at behavioral threshold for cat, it became clear that the audiogram is not governed by stapes displacement, and the writers pointed out the possibilities for contributions from the inner ear and nervous system. Tonndorf and Khanna (1967), however, feel that the middle ear may in fact govern the low-frequency shape of the audiogram. They showed that the fall-off (attributable to the annular ligament) below 600 c/s is −12 dB/octave, i.e., just the slope of the behavioral audiogram, and they pointed out that not only the sound pressure level but the mechano-acoustic power of the sound wave impinging on the eardrum should be considered. This power is said to be the result of multiplying SPL, volume velocity, and the cosine of the phase angle between the two. Volume velocity of the eardrum was estimated either by (1) dividing SPL by acoustic impedance, or (2) by multiplying umbo displacement by effective eardrum area by angular velocity ($2\pi F$). Now when mechano-acoustic power was plotted vs frequency on the same graph as the cat's behavioral audiogram, a somewhat similar slope of reduction for the lower frequencies was seen. The authors therefore concluded that the low-frequency slope of the behavioral audiogram is caused by the middle ear, which is taken to be sensitive to acoustic power, not acoustic pressure alone. Thus the middle ear is looked upon as a power transformer.

Middle-ear dysfunction

The effects on hearing of the absence of structures of the middle ear are known generally to all. In one series of five ears with completely absent middle ear contents, the mean loss through 4 kc/s was about 50 dB. Many types of complications can occur. The whole middle ear can rather suddenly fill with a sero-sanguinous fluid as in aerotitis media (caisson disease), giving a flat loss of about 40 dB at all frequencies. Fluids may cumulate in the tympanum from many other causes, such as head injuries, secretory otitis media and serous otitis media (both of which may turn into mucoid otitis media). Cleft palate children are more prone to mastoid disease often because abnormalities at the base of the skull or palate cause abnormalities of the Eustachian tube, leading to fluid accumulations and increased ear infection.

There may be inequality of static pressure across the eardrum. With

37 Middle-ear dysfunction

an obstructed Eustachian tube, an ear will experience both positive and negative pressures across the eardrum respectively on takeoff and landing in an airplane. Close and Ireland (1961) introduced ± 10 inches water differential static pressure across the eardrum of human subjects, and collected audiograms in an altitude chamber, both at sea level and at simulated 30,000 feet. A positive pressure (eardrum inward) gave hearing losses of about 10 dB at all frequencies; negative pressures (eardrum outward) had progressively less effect at higher frequencies.

The eardrum can also be strongly drawn inward by prolonged contraction of the tensor tympani muscle. Clubb (1965) found the low and middle audiometric frequencies to improve up to 15 dB when the sphenopalatine ganglion in the back of the nose was cocainized (relaxing the tensor tympani). But not only the threshold audiogram was improved: Phonetically-balanced (PB) word discrimination scores were raised by 30 percentage points when a group of 47 patients with strongly retracted eardrums had the tensor tympani muscle tendon cut, and a group of 32 had a cocaine block. This was explained not in terms of improved audiograms of the patients, but as a result of removal of distortion imposed upon the speech by the unnatural eardrum retraction. On one cat, Clubb listened to PB lists through the cochlear microphonic effect; the words were said to become noticeably distorted through the system when the cat's tensor tympani was contracted.

A break in the incudostapedial joint reduces hearing by up to 60 dB. When, however, malleus, incus, and all but the footplate of the stapes are excised, some hearing returns because the structures then no longer exist as a drag on the system to exert attenuation. However, when the middle ear is thus open, sound can impinge upon both oval and round windows simultaneously in phase, thus tending to cancel the effect on the basilar membrane. When this is prevented either by shielding the round window with a septum or by sealing a sound tube over the round window or oval window, the final effect of the middle ear in the cat is seen to be only 20–30 dB across all frequencies (see Wever, Lawrence, and Smith 1948).

Fixation of the ossicular chain is not rare. It can occur congenitally as by an intrusion into the tympanum of the cochlear wall so as to prevent the stapes or incus from moving, or most commonly as a locking of the stapes footplate through an otosclerotic focus. Adhesions binding the ossicles to the tympanum can result from recurrent otitis media and these can be massive enough to depress hearing.

Certain congenital diseases, some with genetic transmission, may affect the middle ear. One of the most dramatic is the Treacher-Collins syndrome; as an autosomal dominant disorder, the symptoms may vary widely from patient to patient, with small mandibles, eye malformations, etc., but especially with small or absent pinnae, complete atresia of the meatus, ossicle malformations or fixations, or reduced tympanum, but often with normal cochlea, which could support normal hearing if surgery were successful in establishing a good conductive path. Another is Van der Hoeve's syndrome, or osteogenesis imperfecta, with lack of proper collagen formation throughout the whole body, in which the ossicles may be malformed, the footplate fused to the promontory, etc. Unfortunately, this disease is often expressed in more or less defective cochleae as well, but at least the middle ear conditions are today generally correctable.

An important caution is that those patients with neural or biochemical lesions in the inner ear or central nervous system, perhaps even genetic and irreversible, may also have progressively deteriorating middle ear disorders. The ears of these patients should not be neglected as hopeless, but should be examined periodically with the otoscope and audiometer. It would be unfair to saddle them with a further, but correctable, condition on top of their other problems.

Reflections on middle-ear physiology

Every aspect of our outer and middle ear has a vital role in our sense of hearing. Pinna, meatus, eardrum, ossicles, muscles, ligaments, joints, bony cavities, and convexities—all are delicately molded and almost perfectly adapted to the work they have to do, of receiving the most minute vibrations of air particles over an efficient range of at least eight octaves in frequency and creating in a fluid column displacements and back-and-forth movements of fluids deep within the head which faithfully mirror the acoustic pressures impinging on the head.

Strenuous efforts to improve on the system have never been successful. If our eardrums were larger, we would not be so omnidirectional; if smaller, our low-tone hearing would suffer. If friction were decreased, our ears would ring to some frequencies and thus reduce our appreciation of clicks and transient sounds generally. If the posterior ligament of the incus were much displaced in any direction, it would be torn off its attachment by the first intense sound. If the Eustachian tube entered the tympanum higher than it does, our ears would cumulate fluid and have a serous conductive loss. If the external meatus were only half as long, the speech-to-noise ratio at one of the most important octaves would suffer by 10 dB. And so on.

Of such a system, poised so surely amid many compromises, we should be especially careful. Children born with unusually small canals or even complete atresia should have the obvious surgery at the first operable moment. An appreciation of the delicate nature of the eardrum would tend to help prevent exposing those in one's charge to inexpert wax removal, pressure changes without precautions for opening the Eustachian tube, swimming in fungus-laden or bacteria-laden water, explosives or even large firecrackers without protection, blows or even slaps to the ear, and (perhaps especially) untreated otitis media. Any infectious process in the tympanum can attack and destroy the bones themselves in time, and much more easily, the gossamer membranes and strands of ligaments. Modern antibiotics have been a godsend in this regard, but in any population, even among younger school children in subsocieties with favorable doctor/population ratios, defective hearing as an aftermath of repeated middle-ear infections is still not at all uncommon; while among other subsocieties, as for example, the Eskimo and American Indian, the problem is very widespread, with sequelae of reduced conductive hearing for the duration of life.

Prevention is of course the watchword. But otologic surgery has made such strides in the past decade or two that no conductive loss today is considered beyond an aggressive attempt to take some positive corrective action. Techniques are now available, for example, to replace the entire contents of the tympanum, with an artificial eardrum, ossicular strut, and artificial footplate.

The cochlea as a hydrodynamic system

The arrangement of structures within the cochlea are shown best by Davis and Associates (1953) (see figure 11). The overall intent is clear, that in- and-out movements of the stapes should induce down-and-up movements respectively of the scala media, rocking on the pivot of the bony spiral lamina, and inducing shear stresses in the hair cells. These stresses arise since the stereocilia are to some extent fixed in the tectorial membrane,

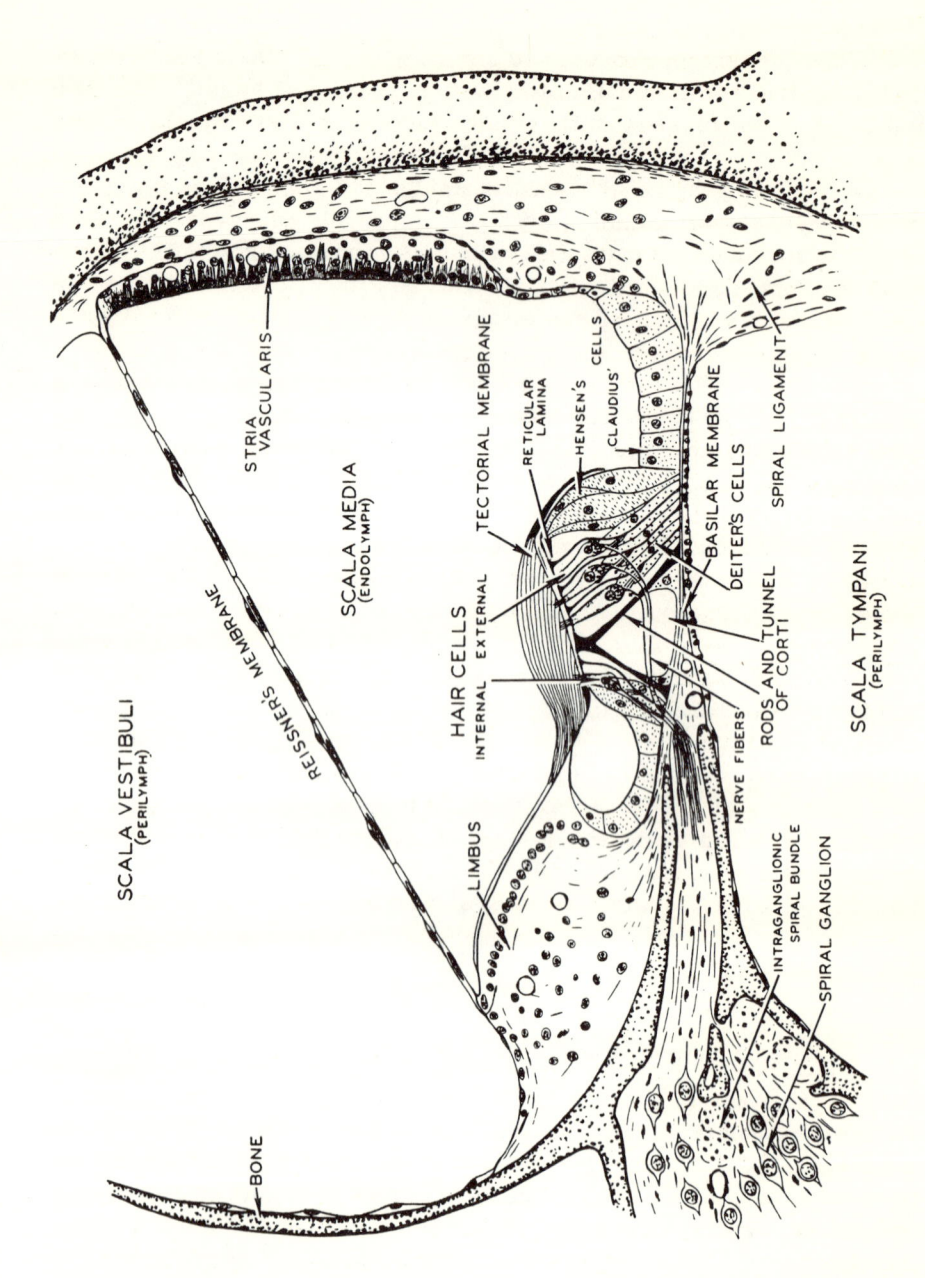

Figure 11 *The structures of the scala media. (Davis and Associates 1953.)*

41 The cochlea as a hydrodynamic system

which has a fulcrum somewhat different from that of the basilar membrane, on which the hair cells sit in their chalices. The hair cells then in some way initiate local excitatory processes in the dendrites of the first-order neurons which closely invest the hair cells, and the neuron ultimately discharges its axon response to the brain stem.

Two broad questions are (1) How can the movements of the scala media, which must be vanishingly small at the threshold of hearing, create enough mechanical shear stress to affect the hair cells and/or their stereocilia? and (2) By what means does the system differentiate among frequencies of stapes oscillation?

It will serve no purpose to recount the older "resonance" theory of Helmholtz, the "telephone" theory of Ewald, etc. These may be found in practically all current summaries of audition, and except as history, fascinating as the story is, they are more misleading than illuminating inasmuch as the points made are today demonstrably incorrect. A theory may in fact be dispensed with if a clear description of what actually occurs is at hand. There follows then an attempt at a descriptive account of cochlear activity, pointing out where information is imprecise and theory must be substituted.

The cochlea as a whole is a hydrodynamic system, and must be understood in those terms. There is a fluid-filled cavity, with a mechanical piston (stapes) capable of exerting alternate inward and outward movements of the fluid next to it. Now as fluids are incompressible, this movement eventuates in movements of a whole column of fluid if the fluid has somewhere to go. There is in fact a pressure release (round window) which (because of Pascal's law which says that pressure at any point in a closed liquid system is transmitted virtually instantaneously to all other points) moves inward and outward synchronously with the stapes (but of course 180° out of phase).

If the cochlear partition (scala media and all its structures) were rigid, when the stapes goes inward, the fluid column would move all in phase, streaming through the helicotrema at the apex of the cochlea, and bulging out the round window. However, indications today are that there exists a shortcut, or shunt. The volume of fluid pushed inward by the stapes, under some conditions of steepness of wavefront and total volume displaced, as shown later on, can more simply displace downward the nearest portion of the cochlear partition, and thus relieve the pressure by pushing the round window outward. This shunt relieves the system of the necessity for displacing the whole volume of fluid in the cochlea to every sound, and largely overcomes the frictional resistance of the tiny helicotrema through which a relatively large amount of fluid would otherwise have to stream very rapidly. In the case of very sharp wavefronts of not very great amplitude (weak high tones) the impedance to the movements of liquid is relatively great, and perhaps only a few millimeters of the cochlear partition are disturbed from equilibrium. In the case of slow wavefronts of high amplitude (loud low tones), the total volume displacement ensures (and the slow build-up of the wavefront makes possible) that a large section of the cochlear partition, perhaps indeed the whole of it, be displaced downward.

According to this view, the cochlear structures are really responsive to the slope, or speed of buildup, of a volume displacement. Thus cochlear analysis is believed to be not essentially in terms of frequency, that is to say, periodicity, but in terms of another aspect of the acoustic wave, the steepness of its wavefront.

Now when the stapes reverses its direction and moves outward, the movements of the fluid column must also reverse themselves. As the stapes withdraws toward its resting position, the reverse effects occur, and restoring forces tend to move the partition upwards toward its resting place.

Hydrodynamic analysis by the cochlea of acoustic frequency The mechanical effects within the cochlea of stapes movement at high sound levels are now fairly clear as the result of observations of Békésy, Tonndorf, and others on human cadavers and cochlear models, and the further analysis of mathematicians and electrical engineers such as Zwislocki and Flanagan.

It is necessary now to describe some of the structural details of the cochlea since they contribute so directly to the activities and sensitivities of hearing.

A seeming paradox is that in the first turn of the cochlea, where all three scalae are largest in cross-section, the basilar membrane is at its narrowest. It widens irregularly by a factor of about five as it unrolls to the apex of the cochlea. The effect of width, together with other conditions such as the larger diameter of the fibers of the basilar membrane at the apex, and their differential loading by other cells, is to reduce the stiffness of the membrane about 100 times (i.e., 40 dB) along the basal-apical gradient. No other aspect of the cochlear partition varies by this much. Now when the stapes pushes inward with a slow thrust, let us say within 10 msec (equivalent to the time between the resting condition and the

43 The cochlea as a hydrodynamic system

maximum condensation condition of a 25 c/s acoustic wave in the ear canal), the pressures within the fluids are transmitted within 0.025 msec or less (the speed of sound in salt water) to all parts of the cochlea and vestibule. But the rather stiff basilar membrane is not depressed, because the mass of fluid moved by the stapes, and the friction due to the walls and helicotrema, are not so great but that little resistance is offered to this slow movement from base to apex of the perilymph in scala vestibuli, and from apex to base of the perilymph in scala tympani. Consequently, the perilymph streams through the helicotrema and bulges out the round window. Of course, as the stapes swings back, the perilymph is pulled back through the helicotrema again for the next 20 msec, to the maximum outward position of the stapes (acoustic rarefaction in the external meatus), while the round window bulges inward. And so on.

Now let us suppose a 250 c/s tone. The inward motion of the stapes lasts only 1 msec, much too fast for the perilymph, on account of its mass and the friction, to stream through the helicotrema. The inward displacement of the stapes would therefore be sharply reduced at 250 c/s unless a shunt could be found reducing the mass and friction to be overcome. The cochlear partition—particularly the basilar membrane—provides this shunt. Its stiffness, and the fluid mass involved, are not so great but that a one-msec thrust inward of the stapes will displace most of the partition downward, equalizing pressure through the round window, and leaving untroubled the perilymph at and near the helicotrema.

For a 2500 c/s tone, with an inward thrust lasting only 0.1 msec, the stiffness and mass are so great that the shunt must be provided by the first part of the cochlear partition up to about its middle, and half the perilymph column is unmoved.

For a 25,000 c/s tone, with a thrust inward lasting only 0.01 msec, the fluid presents such a load that the stapes motion is impeded completely, virtually no perilymph is moved, and we are effectively deaf to that frequency.

Thus there exists a frequency-dependent gradient up the cochlea, the highest audible tone stimulating only the basal end, lower tones stimulating all the membrane up to a point distant from the stapes depending upon frequency.

As the stimulating tone increases in intensity, the stapes goes in farther, but of course with the same timing. More fluid is displaced, and the basilar membrane is correspondingly more active, but the maximum position on the membrane of the frequency gradient is not appreciably shifted.

44 Anatomy and physiology of peripheral hearing mechanism

Frequency layout in the cochlea The frequency layout of the cochlea has been exhaustively studied, and dozens of graphs have been published relating frequency to distance from the stapes. Figure 12 is a recent one incorporating data from stimulation deafness and electrophysiological studies. It can be assumed that the layouts in cat and man are very similar. This figure shows that some uncertainty still exists in the layout for the lowest octaves, where place along the membrane may not be the dominant cue for pitch.

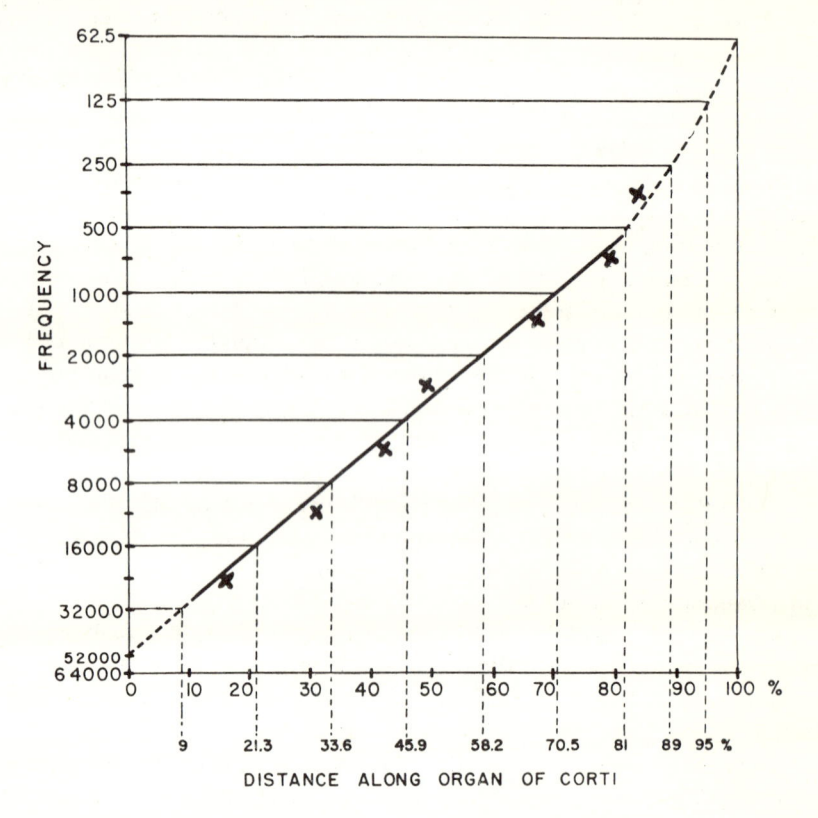

Figure 12 *Frequency map of the cochlea. (Schuknecht 1960.)*

Pattern of deformation of the cochlear partition The exact shape of the deformation of the basilar membrane at any instant is somewhat uncertain. We can dismiss at once any notion of a free traveling wave, in the sense of a wave traveling up a rope when one end is snapped. Once the stapes and fluid column have reached their inmost position, and the stapes begins outward motion, at that instant the fluid column must of necessity reverse its direction and the basilar membrane start its upward motion. The motion of the stapes and of the basilar membrane at all points up to the point of maximum displacement are essentially in phase. Thus virtually all motions of fluids and structures within the cochlea are forced by the stapes, and do not proceed to move under energetics of their own. This does not mean of course that the *patterns* of such motions are not governed by the details of the intracochlear structures. There is the further fact that motion of the basilar membrane at points more apical than that of maximum displacement begin to lag the stapes in phase, and are in that sense free, but these displacements decline to zero very quickly both in time and distance, and probably have little to do with the process of hearing.

A four-dimensional picture of basilar membrane deformation over time can best be built up in one's mind by contemplating the pictures drawn by Békésy (1960) (see his widely-reproduced figures 11-20 and 11-49) of movement produced in the cadaver under very strong acoustic stimulation and actually seen by him under stroboscopic illumination. These are to be compared with electrophysiological data from Teas, Eldredge, and Davis (1962) figure 13 and Legouix (1966) figure 14 in the guinea pig. It is clear that each frequency generates its maximum movement at a certain region of the basilar membrane, but that a considerable extent of the membrane is also engaged, particularly for low tones. An intense low tone may deform a large portion of the membrane from the basal end to the point of maximum amplitude, but apicalward from this point the deformation falls to nothing within a very few millimeters (this is a basic reason why low tones generally mask higher tones, but higher tones have little effect on the lower.)

Tasaki, Davis, and Legouix (1952) and Legouix (1966) have shown that this deformation follows a time course. As the stapes moves inward, the fluid column first depresses the membrane at the first or most basal part of the final deformation pattern, and the deformation proceeds upward to its most apicalward extent, reaching its maximum distance from the stapes with some phase lag when the stapes has reached its most inward position. Legouix shows a progressive slowing of the speed of deformation from an initial 4 mm/sec to only 0.3 mm/sec (see figure 15).

Thus, as the stapes moves inward, a form of traveling wave moves upward, its phase governed by (though not exactly identical with) that of the stapes, and its three-dimensional pattern determined by the mass, stiffness,

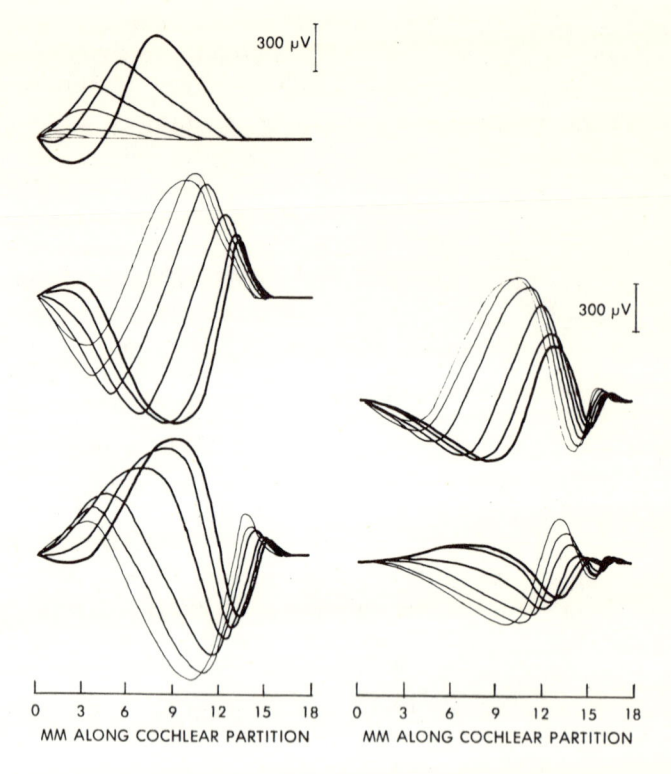

46 Anatomy and physiology of peripheral hearing mechanism

Figure 13 *Successive positions of basilar membrane displacement. Instantaneous cochlear-microphonic voltage as a function of distance along the cochlear partition at 0.1-msec. intervals. Thicker lines represent more recent times. The progression from the top left to the bottom set on the right is a continuous sequence. Between sets go from the thickest line in the set above to the thinnest line in the set below. The signal for this figure was almost the same as the 1.05-msec transient. (Teas, Eldredge, and Davis 1962.)*

and friction of the intracochlear structures.

The possibility of non-mechanical stimulation Another quite different type of cochlear action has been suggested at least for weaker sound intensities. As has been mentioned, the amplitude of the stapes at audiometric threshold is of the order of 10^{-11} cm, something like less than one billionth of an inch, and of the basilar membrane an equally almost unbelievable dimension as a mechanical driving force. Many writers have

47 The cochlea as a hydrodynamic system

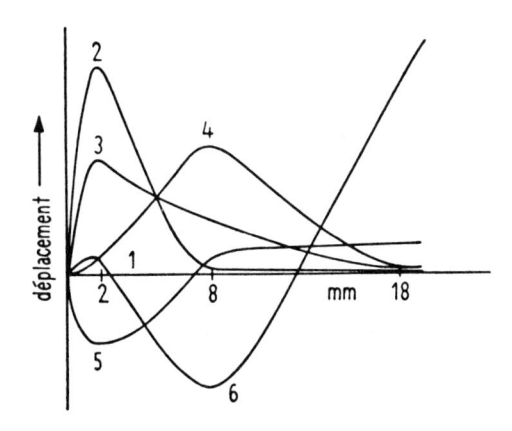

Figure 14 *Successive positions of basilar membrane displacement in response to an acoustic click. Displacement is relative; ordinate is distance in mm from the stapes. (Legouix 1966.)*

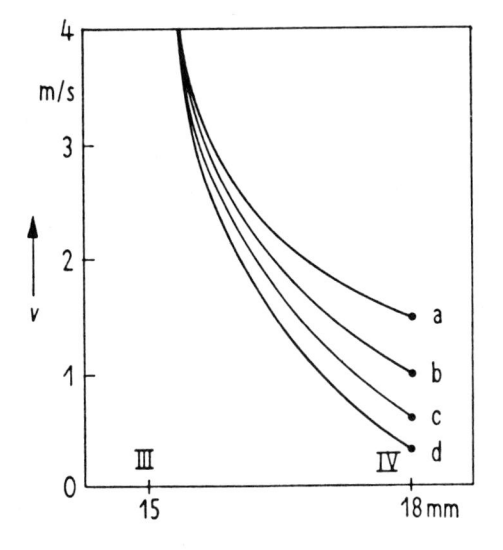

Figure 15 *Speed of cochlear wave. V: velocity in meters per second; a: speed of first wave; b–d: speed of successive waves; III: third cochlear turn in guinea pig; IV: fourth turn in guinea pig. (Legouix 1966.)*

pointed out the seeming impossibility of shear stress acting upon a cell with such vanishingly small mechanical movement. As one possibility, Naftalin (1967, 1968) has shown in a model of the cochlea consisting simply of fluid in a truncated pyramid that foci of high frequencies may be induced at the basal end of the pyramid, and of low frequencies at the apical end. These were shown not to be simply standing waves, and it was found that their sharpness could be increased by adding a septum simulating the basilar membrane. Thus the cochlea may analyze frequency by virtue solely of its geometric construction, in the absence perhaps of any shear stress whatever on the basilar membrane. The smaller mechanical movements of the stapes would not then create shear stresses, but initiate an acoustic wave in the fluids of the cochlea, and this acoustic wave would be analyzed by the geometry of the cochlea. Some support for this theory comes from the fact that the speed of sound in a gel, such as that of the tectorial membrane, is only about 5 mm/msec, just the time order of Békésy's supposed mechanical traveling wave. The speed of the acoustic wave then, rather than the traveling wave, could create the condition of the tapped time-delay line in the cochlea. Whether Naftalin's theory is proved correct or not, there is certainly no reason why the ear may not have adopted two quite distinct systems of analysis, one for weak and one for stronger stimulation. Such arrangements are not unknown in the sensorium generally.

Bone conduction When the skull vibrates at sonic frequencies, the acoustic energies are transmitted to the fluids of the cochlea; the result is a sensation of hearing. But here the ossicular chain is not primarily involved, and the foregoing considerations based upon stapes movement do not tell the whole story. Bone conducted hearing is a fascinating chapter in its own right, and an understanding of how the cochlea analyzes frequency by other routes is basic to our understanding of the whole inner ear mechanism. One asks (1) in the case of airborne sound, how this energy is picked up by the skull, and (2) how the cochlea receives and analyzes this energy.

1. *Movements of the skull in response to sound* Békésy (1960) placed a bone-conduction vibrator on the forehead of subjects, applying a constant force of 250 g, and measured the amplitude of vibration of the skull with a probe sensitive to 10^{-5} cm. He found that at 800 c/s the (extrapolated) movement at human threshold was about 3×10^{-10} cm, later amending this to 6×10^{-10} cm at 3 kc/s. This amplitude of vibration of the whole skull at threshold is of the order of magnitude of the displacement of each air particle (and of the eardrum and stapes) at a pressure equal to the threshold of airborne hearing at 3 kc/s. Figure 16 shows some of these relations. It would seem that the same particle displacement within the cochlear fluids yields behavioral threshold whether these displacements are engendered by the stapes in the usual route or by the skull in the bc (bone conduction) route.

49 The cochlea as a hydrodynamic system

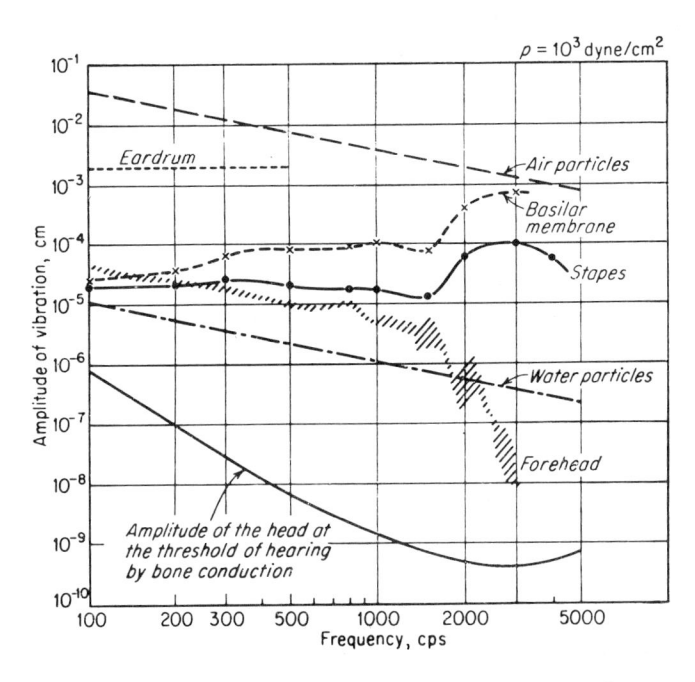

Figure 16 *Upper six curves, amplitudes of vibration of the human head, eardrum, stapes, basilar membrane, and air and water particles for a sound pressure of 10^3 dynes per sq cm. Lowermost curve, amplitude of the head at the threshold of hearing by bone conduction. (Békésy 1960.)*

The skull will also vibrate in response to airborne sound. Békésy (1960) placed a man in a free field 114 dB over threshold by air conduction, at 1 kc/s, and measured the amplitude of motion of a front tooth, using a special pickup very sensitive to vibration but very insensitive to airborne sound. At 3 kc/s, the skull movement was 10^{-8} cm (extrapolated down to 2×10^{-14} cm at airborne threshold). It appears that for frequencies of 1.5 kc/s and lower, airborne sound is about 60 dB more effective than bone-conducted sound.

2. *Routes for vibratory energy to reach the cochlea* (a) Compressional route. Below its resonant frequency (1.8 kc/s) the whole skull moves in a translational wave in one direction, then the other, in phase with the applied force; but at about 1.5 kc/s, as the forehead goes backward the back of the head goes foreward, and vice versa, introducing compression in the

front-back direction; so that at 1.5 kc/s and especially at higher frequencies, waves are propagated through the skull setting up very complex translational and compressional patterns.

The waves transmitted through the skull would have no influence on cochlear mechanics, and hence none on hearing, if the displacements were equal on both sides of the basilar membrane. However, the action of the round window is much more mobile than the release of pressure through the oval window, with its brake of the annular ligament and ossicles, and thus through this asymmetry the basilar membrane undergoes motion.

Békésy (1960) showed that with an open external meatus, increasing the air pressure in the meatus (by way of a large box applied to the side of the head) had a 10 dB greater effect on air conduction (ac) than on bone conduction (bc) thresholds. From this he inferred that the compressional route is of much reduced importance in bc hearing with open meatus.

(b) *Inertial route.* A second route for vibratory energy to reach the cochlea by bc is by way of the inertia of the ossicles. As the skull is moved, the ossicles tend by their mass not to move, and thus the cochlea moves relative to the footplate. This of course has the same effect as when the footplate moves relative to the cochlea.

(c) *An ac route through the external ear canal.* A third route is the ensonification of the air in the external ear canal by way of skull vibrations. With the meatus open, the sound leak to the outside renders this route negligible, but with the meatus stoppled as by a forefinger or earplug, the route is important. As Békésy (1960) showed, the effects on ac and bc thresholds were the same when with a closed meatus the ossicular chain was relatively immobilized by increasing the air pressure in the external meatus. This shows that hearing by bc with a closed meatus is largely through this route. The strong contribution of this third route with the meatus closed can be estimated from the occlusion effect: bc thresholds with open meatus and with the meatus closed by the finger are compared. In the latter case, an improvement in bc threshold by 10–15 dB exists, about the same for all low frequencies; but the improvement reduces as the resonance of the ossicles is approached, and is effectively zero at 2 kc/s and above. No such occlusion effect is seen in a patient with a complete actual or effective loss of the middle ear.

(d) *An ac route through the round window.* A fourth route is by way of vibratory energy ensonifying the air in the middle ear. This route could be of some importance in underwater hearing where the air in the external canal is replaced with water, and the ossicles loaded, or under pressure, so that they are not free to move. Intense sound energy in the small air bubble in the tympanum would be expected to transmit energy through the round window with an efficiency much greater than the 30-dB loss at the usual air-water interface. The relative contribution of this route has not been established.

One may conclude that under certain conditions of stimulation—airborne, waterborne, or direct vibratory, with either a large or small volume of air in the external meatus, or no air at all—the major role of energy transfer in each case will be assumed by one or other route of the four possible ones.

Frequency analysis in the cochlea No matter how acoustic energy reaches the cochlea, whether from the usual ac route, or one or more of the bc routes, or whatever the relative contribution of all active routes in any particular situation, the cochlea analyzes the input spectrum in the identical fashion. Lowy (1942) found that both ac and bc energy, suitably balanced in intensity and phase, could reduce movement of the basilar membrane to zero. One must conclude that the identical hair cells respond to the maximum effect of either ac or bc energy at any frequency.

Wever and Lawrence (1952) led sound to the cat cochlea simultaneously by a tube sealed over the stapes and by another tube sealed over a hole in the apex of the cochlea. An electrode was placed on the base and another on the apex of the cochlea. The electricity generated by the hair cells on the basilar membrane (referred to as the cochlear microphonic [CM]) and picked up by this electrode arrangement is a measure of basilar membrane movement (see p. 60 below). The CM is a rather exact simulation by electricity of the frequency, phase, and intensity of the acoustic event at the eardrum and is a valuable tool for studying cochlear activity. It is often called the Wever-Bray phenomenon after its discoverers. In this case, the cochlear microphonic at either electrode could always be reduced to zero in response to any frequency, or amplified to twice the magnitude from a single input, by controlling the stimulus intensity and phase. Thus the pattern of stimulation of the hair cells is the same no matter where the sound is introduced.

This crucial experiment and its ingenious controls bears upon the way in which the cochlea analyzes the frequency of a stimulus. Evidently the two stimuli, basal and apical, do not simply set up traveling waves originating at the sound inputs and moving in opposite directions, as all traveling wave theories predict. Neither does the apical wave simply move toward the stapes at the speed of sound and then create a basal-apicalward traveling wave at a much slower speed, as Fletcher (1951) once assumed. The simplest explanation is that of Wever and Lawrence (1954) who credit Fletcher with the initial assumption, that a traveling wave, in the sense of a propagated wave traveling slowly by way of a mechanical coupling of neighboring strands on the basilar membrane, is not really created at all, but that the relatively uncoupled elements of the membrane respond, each to its own frequency, as soon as the acoustic wave impinges upon it.

Wever's and Lawrence's determination of the speed of effects through the cochlea rests upon their demonstration that the apical-basal sources create in-phase conditions at both basal and apical electrodes for all frequencies of 1 kc/s and below, and phase changes of only 35° at 10 kc/s (a time delay of only 0.012 msec).

These data on cat have been somewhat superseded by those of Tasaki, Davis, and Legouix (1952) on the guinea pig, where the whole cochlea was available for electrode placement. Here the basal-apical progression was found to be somewhat slower, of the order of 2.5 msec—inconsistent with the speed of sound in perilymph and consistent with Békésy's traveling wave theory. For the front of a single pressure wave passing up the cochlea, Legouix (1966) found a delay as long as 4 msec for the guinea pig.

The cochlear electricities

Perilymph direct current (DC) A small electrode inserted in the perilymph near the stapes, and another inserted at points up the cochlear canals, reveals a distribution of constant DC potential differences amounting to a maximum of 3 millivolts (mV) at the helicotrema (see figure 17). Since the perilymph is chemically homogeneous, this must indicate a constant DC flow inside the cochlea. If now a sound activates the stapes, the DC charge at any point drops immediately to a lesser plateau, the amount of the drop being proportional to sound intensity; and it returns immediately when the sound is turned off. If the sound is very loud but not loud enough to cause a decline over time in the cochlear microphonic, the drop in DC nevertheless increases as long as the sound is on, and takes an appreciable time to recover when the sound is turned off. In one such experiment, when the tone was turned on, the DC dropped immediately by 0.9 mV, and gradually over 10 sec by another 0.11 mV, then required 8 msec to recover

53 The cochlear electricities

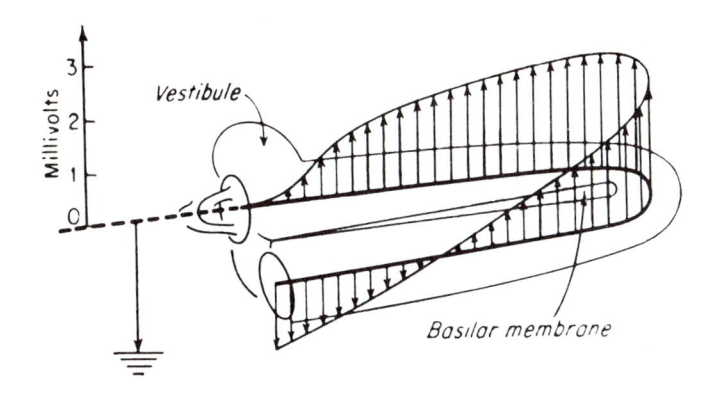

Figure 17 *Direct current potentials in the perilymph of the vestibular and tympanic scalae. (Békésy 1960.)*

when the sound was turned off. The perilymph DC is very sensitive to lack of oxygen.

It was these DC potentials which Békésy used to prove that the generation of energy involved in hearing does not come from the mechanical energy of the acoustic stimulus, but from the metabolism of the body: when a thin glass rod depressed the basilar membrane, the DC voltage in the scala tympani near the round window became more positive, and continued to do so for the 10 minutes of the depression. Here the mechanical work done by the glass rod ceases as soon as the movement ceases, but the electrical work continues indefinitely to cumulate. Békésy calculated that it exceeded the mechanical work performed after about 1 second of depression.

Positive and negative endocochlear potentials (+EP, −EP) Békésy (1960) was the first to explore the DC pools within the scala media (see figure 18). Relative to scala vestibuli, a negativity of −20 mV appeared as the electrode punctured Reissner's membrane at a point halfway up the scalae, increased to +50 mV throughout the endolymph, and dropped to −40 mV in the organ of Corti. Potentials of as much as +80 mV were found in the basal turn. These +80 mV potentials have been called the endocochlear potentials (+EP).

The potentials of −40 mV in the organ of Corti were assumed by Békésy and later workers (Tasaki and Fernàndez 1952; Tasaki, Davis, and

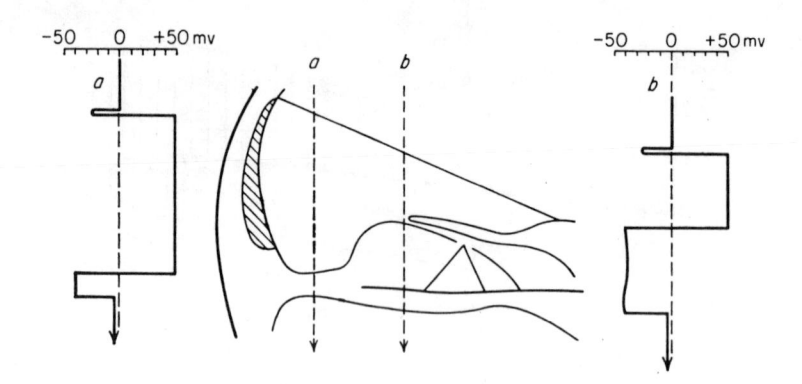

Figure 18 *Changes in the DC potential during a downward movement of the electrode at two positions as shown. (Békésy 1960.)*

Eldredge 1954) to be intracellular, but more recently they have been found as large as −80 mV and are generally distributed throughout all the fluids and areas between the basilar membrane and the tectorial membrane (thus giving rise to the notion of a third cochlear fluid, the Cortilymph). Békésy showed that −EP existed also in the stria vascularis (see figure 11).

Lawrence (1967) showed that the tectorial membrane was a completely insulating tissue, of quite neutral charge, between the +EP of the endolymph and the −EP of the Cortilymph. Thus the DC potential difference between the endolymph and the body of any hair cell, including the cuticular surface and all of the stereocilia except those tips embedded in the tectorial membrane, can equal the algebraic sum of −80 plus +80 mV, or 1/6 of a volt, a large charge indeed.

The significance of this pool of DC energy, or battery, is not at present clear in view of the prevailing ascendancy of the chemical theory of dendritic stimulation. The electrical current flow would seem to arise in the stria vascularis, since that tissue is heavily supplied with blood vessels and nutrients, and to proceed through the organ of Corti, where it could be modified by action of the hair cells. The cochlear microphonic could then be regarded as a ripple on the strong DC charge.

These electrical arrangements and processes are of course accompanied and undergirded by biochemical conditions and the equations of metabolism and catabolism; in no other instance in the body do electrical or chemical events exist one without the other. But the cogency of a 0.16V battery, and a region of variable resistance controlling its flow, much in the pattern of the vacuum tube where a microvolt can modulate the behavior of an immensely larger charge, is such that the writer would one day be extremely surprised should a definitive experiment establish the electrical events as only an inconsiderable moiety of the whole.

+EP is maintained by metabolism of the stria vascularis (Tasaki and Spyropoulos 1959), but it does not depend on ionic content in any simple way, since the endolymph (high in K, low in Na) can be replaced by perilymph (low in K, high in Na) without affecting +EP (Tasaki and Fernàndez 1952). That the −EP is maintained by the basilar membrane is shown by the fact that concentrations of NaCl (Wever and Bray 1937) and KCl (Tasaki and Fernàndez 1952) in the scala tympani quickly destroy the cochlear microphonic, *and likewise the* −EP in the organ of Corti (Butler 1965, Lawrence 1967).

The relation between +EP and the cochlear microphonic was demonstrated by Konishi, Kelsey, and Singleton (1967) in anoxic (deprived of oxygen) guinea pigs: when DC current was passed between scala media and scala tympani so as to render EP more positive or negative, the cochlear microphonic was increased and decreased respectively. However, though they may often covary, the mechanism whereby the EP is modulated (i.e., the cochlear microphonic) may be quite different from the mechanism of *generation* of the EP.

The hair cells and the cochlear microphonic It is obvious from gross anatomy that the more radial side of the basilar membrane will move more than the more central side for a certain depression of scala media, and that very slight movements might not affect the more central side at all. Let us examine what use is made of this construction. The basilar membrane contains the supporting tunnel of Corti, a structure based upon an arch of two rigid cells, bound tightly together at the top like two clasped hands, their bases firmly fixed apart on the basilar membrane (see figure 11). The two rows of cells form a spiral tunnel running the length of the basilar membrane. On the inner side runs a single row of hair cells, about 3500 (2800–4400) in the human ear, and on the outer side three or four rows of hair cells, about 13,400 (11,200–16,000) (see Bredberg 1968). The more numerous outer hair cells, being on the more movable portion of the membrane should be responsive to slighter movements (see figure 19).

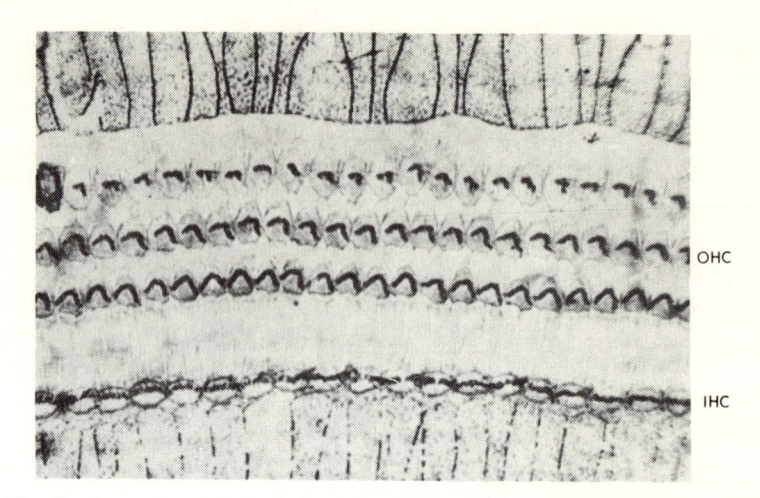

56 Anatomy and physiology of peripheral hearing mechanism

Figure 19 *Surface view of the hair cells of the guinea pig cochlea, upper turn. Note the three rows of outer hair cells (OHC) with their W-shaped stereocilia, and the single row of inner hair cells (IHC) with their stereocilia in parallel lines. (Katagiri et al 1968.)*

The inner hair cells are more tenpin-shaped than the cylindrical outer cells (see figure 20). Outer hair cells in the first row nearest the arch of Corti are shortest, and longest in the outside row (see figure 21). Each hair cell is held firmly as in a chalice by a Dieter's cell, allowing free access for nerve endings to the base of the hair cell.

Although the number of inner hair cells along the basilar membrane is about the same (about 100) per mm distance from base to apex, the number of outer hair cells increases from 300 per mm at the base to about 500 per mm at the apex. However, the basilar membrane widens from 0.1 to 0.5 mm and the distance between adjacent outer hair cells also becomes large, so that the density of cells actually decreases from about 155 per 0.01 sq mm at the base to only 90 per 0.01 sq mm at 1.5 turns up the cochlea (Bredberg 1968). Probably the feature of geometry which is most important is the density per length rather than per area.

Figure 20 *The inner hair cell (upper diagram) and the outer hair cell (lower diagram). D: the Dieter's cell cup in which the outer hair cell rests; H: hairs, or stereocilia; NE_1: type I (afferent) nerve ending; NE_2: type II (efferent) nerve ending; B: basal body; PM: plasma membrane; Nu: nucleus; RM: reticular membrane; UP: the phalangeal process of the Dieter's cell which reaches to the reticular membrane. (Spoendlin 1967.)*

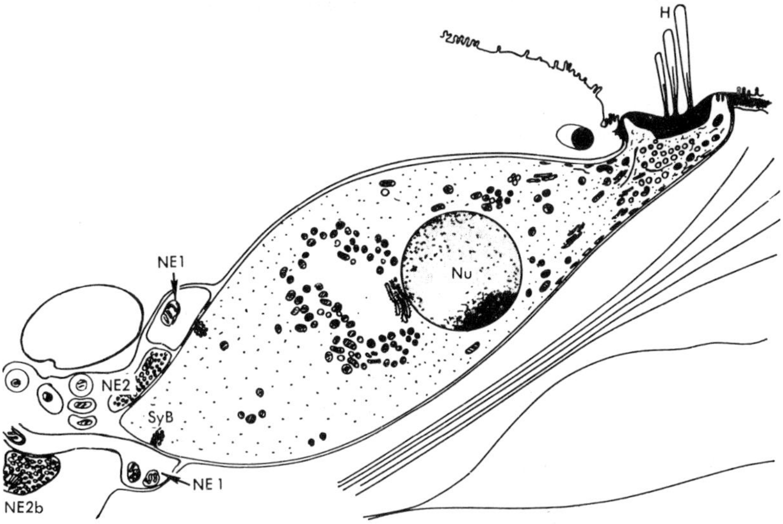
H
NE1
Nu
NE2
SyB
NE 1
NE2b

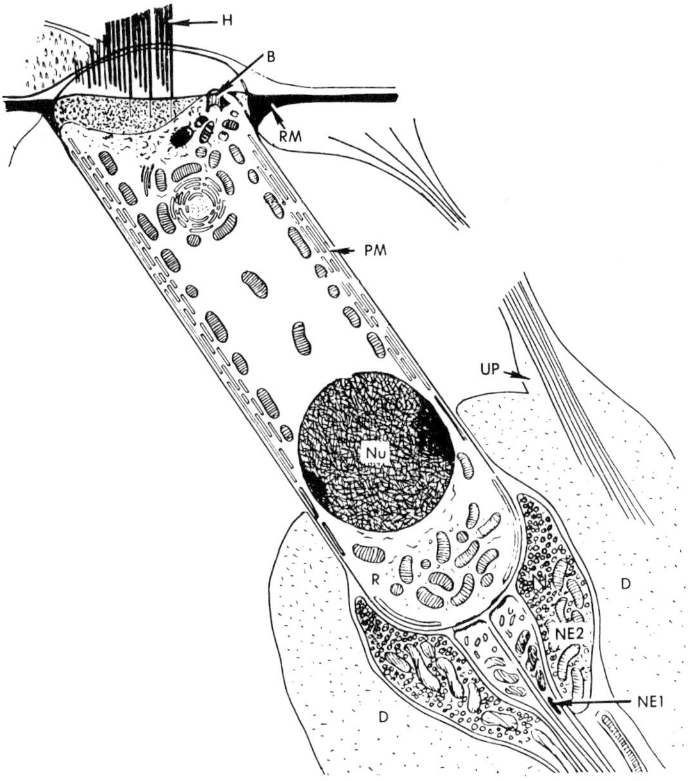
H
B
RM
PM
UP
Nu
R
D
NE2
NE1
D

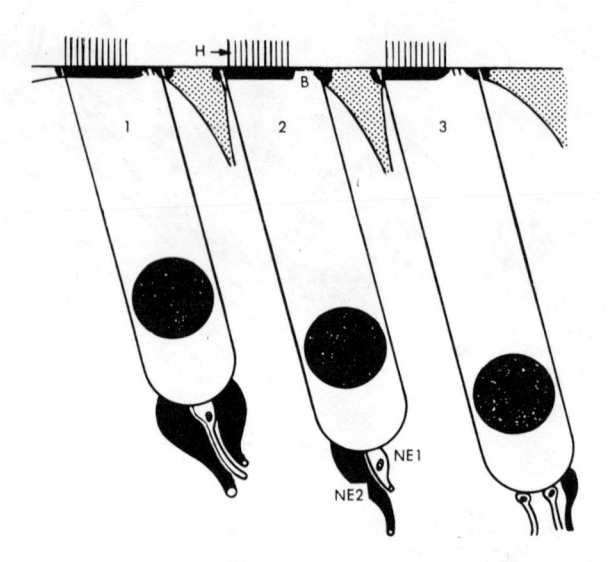

Figure 21 *Variations in the outer hair cells. Apical half, guinea pig cochlea. 1: cell from innermost row; 2: a middle-row cell; 3: cell from outermost row. Rows differ in cell volume and in extent of contact with nerves. NE_1: afferent ending; NE_2: efferent ending; H: hairs or stereocilia; B: basal body. (Engstrom, Ades, and Andersson 1966.)*

The upper ends of the hair cells are supported rigidly by a structure, the reticular lamina, looking like a piece of swiss cheese. Each hole in the reticular lamina is filled with the upper end of a hair cell. The lamina moves with the basilar membrane as a unit when the scala media moves, so that the body of the hair cell is not itself subjected to any appreciable shear stress.

The stereocilia are not, however, thus supported. These are very numerous, 60–120 per cell, rather stiff, and shaped in a triple W, open toward the modiolus (see figures 19 and 22). The cilia at the ends of the arms of the W are longer than those in the angles. Only about 1/5 of the stereocilium is inserted into the cuticular surface of the hair cell (see figure 22A). The longer ciliar tips of at least the outer hair cells are embedded lightly in the under surface of the tectorial membrane. This membrane is held firmly by the lip of the spiral osseous lamina, but more radially it floats freely in the endolymph. It is a rather thick, broad, heavy sheet which must possess considerable inertia and, at rest, must lie rather heavily on the cilia. It is perhaps to support this dead weight that so many cilia are found per cell;

59   The cochlear electricities

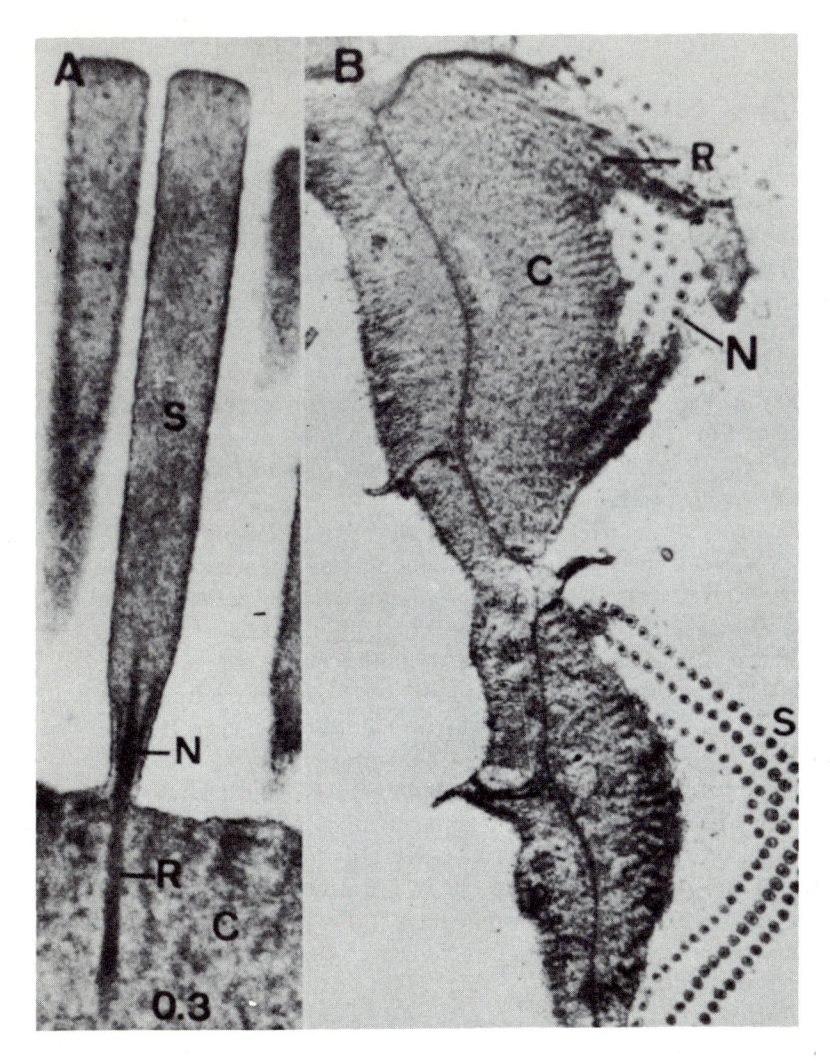

Figure 22   *The stereocilia. Print A shows a longitudinal section through one sensory hair (S) with its flattened upper end; the narrow neck portion (N), and the rootlet (R) which penetrates into the cuticular plate (C). Print B shows a horizontal section through the surface area of two outer hair cells with the cuticular plate (C) and the sensory hairs (S) arranged in typical W pattern. The rootlets of the hairs (R) are clearly seen within the cuticular plate surrounded by a lighter zone (the rootlet canal). In the neck portion of the stereocilium (N), just above the cell surface, a dark central core is surrounded by a lighter zone. (Spoendlin 1966.)*

too few cilia might be crushed by its mass. Also, the different lengths of the cilia insure that some of them, no matter what the state of mechanical activity of the system, will be stimulated by another increment of movement.

We see by now two of the several different mechanisms existing to extend the dynamic range of intensities over which the ears can give differential loudness response: a graded degree of movement from the innermost to the outermost rows of hair cells, and a graded activation of the longest to the shortest stereocilia.

The mechanisms whereby the hair cells stimulate the dendrites is not known. It is known that acoustic stimulation is followed with little or no latency, except for the time delay of the traveling wave, by the appearance of the ac CM at the cuticular surface of the hair cells (it is most likely true that this is the case only for the outer hair cells—it is not established that the inner cells produce CM).

CM was at one time thought by Wever to be a change in the ion charge across the cell membrane when the cell was sheared; but the extremely minute movements of the basilar membrane, already referred to above (at behavioral threshold the supposed movements of the basilar membrane are 10^{-11} cm, whereas the diameter of the stereocilium [10^{-5} cm] is 100,000 times greater), and the rigid support of the hair cell at both ends, render it unlikely that, at least at threshold of hearing, the cell itself has sheared. It seems more likely that deformations of the tallest stereocilia in response to the faintest audible sound, act as a trigger, or mechano-electrical transducer, to initiate an electrochemical event in the hair cell. There are vertical striations within the cilia, and horizontal structures in the body of the hair cell, reminiscent of a battery, and a specialized portion near the top of the cell toward which the W of the stereocilia is oriented (analogous to the kinocilium of the labyrinth), the functions of which are at present unclear.

Tasaki, Davis, and Eldredge (1954) showed that the CM was indeed generated at the hair-bearing end of the hair cell, and felt that the CM represents ac current flow as the transmembrane resistance changes as a result of movements of the stereocilia.

Negative and positive summating potentials (−SP, +SP) A puzzling phenomenon is a negative DC shift in the CM at moderate and louder sound intensities (the so-called negative summating potential, −SP, of Davis, Fernàndez, and McAuliffe (1950). Davis (1960) suggested that the tectorial membrane undergoes a steady one-way movement in a basal-apical direction at these intensities, which could bend the hairs in this direction and give rise to a DC potential of the inner hair cells. At that time, a positive phase of SP was known but was not incorporated into Davis's theory. Johnstone and Johnstone (1965) proposed that a negative SP was generated at weak intensities by outer hair cells, but changed to a positive SP generated at moderate and loud intensities by inner hair cells. However, SP occurs in the avian cochlea where no differentiation of inner and outer hair cells exists. Kupperman (1966) showed that +SP starts simultaneously with CM (has no latency or threshold) and reasoned that it is the consequence of a "leakage current" through the organ of Corti; while the —SP has a latency equal to the action potential of the nerve, and is the summated effect of the asynchronous action potentials.

Whitfield and Ross offer the simplest explanation. They pointed out that the motion of the basilar membrane is by no means symmetrical about its resting position, and that a DC component of the ac CM could arise, greater as the asymmetry increased, either with increasing acoustic intensities or artificially as is found with induced changes of fluid pressures across the scala media.

In any case, there is now little support for the theory that the SP is a form of electricity which participates directly in the stimulation of the dendrite.

The Kiang-Peake "slow potential" In an ear with nerve VIII cut, degeneration of the whole nerve fibers eventually occurs and the electrical output of the ear is presumably then due exclusively to the hair cells (Rawdon-Smith and Hawkins 1939). In such an ear Kiang and Peake (1960) found that when CM was subtracted by averaging over many condensation and rarefaction clicks, there still remained a slow DC potential in response even to weak sound intensities. It was noted that this might be the +SP of Davis, but it appeared at SPLs too low to produce +SP, and its latency was about 0.4 msec longer; and the authors suggested that it may be an intracochlear event over and above CM, +SP, and —SP which might in fact initiate neural events when other precursors were ineffective.

Cochlear after-potential Stopp (1967) with an electrode in the scala media discovered another positive potential in the mammalian and avian cochlea. This potential arises after an acoustic event terminates, and is opposite in polarity to SP. Its magnitude and duration depend on the duration of the acoustic event and it looks much like a neuron's after-potential found after a train of nerve impulses has occurred. Panayiotopoulos and Stopp (1968) showed that it is highly dependent upon Na in the perilymph: when only 10% of the Na in the perilymph was removed, the positive after-potential was abolished, but it returned when the normal Na in the perilymph was re-established. SP usually seen at the onset of stimulation was not changed with removal of all Na from the perilymph. Evidently the cochlear after-potential and SP have different generative mechanisms; Panayiotopoulos and Stopp feel that the experiments with Na and the chemical complex DNP point to the possible generation of the cochlear after-potential by an ionic mechanism in the hair cells similar to that in the neuron, rather than to the accumulation of a chemical transmitter at the hair cell-dendrite junction.

This volume has led the reader through the peripheral auditory system from pinna to cochlea. As the next step in the study of hearing he should approach the topic of how the auditory nervous system codes and decodes the electrical analogue of acoustic events.

References

ANDERSON, H. C.; HANSEN, C. C.; and NEERGAARD, E. B. 1964. Experimental studies on sound transmission in the human ear. II *Acta Otolaryngologica* 56: 307–317.

ANSON, B. J., and DONALDSON, J. A. 1967. *The Surgical Anatomy of the Temporal Bone and Ear.* Philadelphia: W. B. Saunders.

ANSON, B. J.; HARPER, D. G.; and WINCH, T. R. 1964. Intra-osseous blood supply of the auditory ossicles in man. *Annals of Otology, Rhinology and Laryngology* 73: 645–658.

BATTEAU, D. W. 1967. The role of the pinna in human localization. *Proceedings of the Royal Society of Medicine* 168, Series B: 158–180.

BÉKÉSY, G. V. 1960. *Experiments in hearing.* Trans. and ed. E. G. Wever. New York: McGraw-Hill.

BORG, E. 1968. A quantitative study of the effect of the acoustical stapedius reflex on sound transmission through the middle ear of man. *Acta Otolaryngologica* 66: 461–472.

BREDBERG, G. 1968. Cellular pattern and nerve supply of the human organ of Corti. *Acta Otolaryngologica, Supplement* 236: 135.

BUTLER, R. A. 1965. Some experimental observations on the DC resting potential in the guinea-pig cochlea. *Journal of the Acoustical Society of America* 37: 429–433.

CLOSE, P., and IRELAND, R. G. 1961. Alterations in the pure tone threshold following changes in both absolute and differential pressures upon the ear. *Journal of Auditory Research* 1: 194–201.

CLUBB, R. W. 1965. Discrimination improvement. *Laryngoscope* 75: 939–945.

DAHMANN, H. 1929. Zur physiologie des Hörens. *Z. Hals Nas.-Ohrenheilk.* 24: 462–497.

DALLOS, P. S. 1964. Dynamics of the acoustic reflex: phenomenological aspects. *Journal of the Acoustical Society of America*: 2175–2183.

DAVIS, H. 1960. Mechanisms of excitation of auditory nerve impulses. Ch. 2 in *Neural Mechanisms of the Auditory and Vestibular Systems.* G. L. Rasmussen and W. F. Windle, eds. Springfield, Ill.: C. C. Thomas.

────── and Associates. 1953. Acoustic trauma in the guinea pig. *Journal of the Acoustical Society of America* 25: 1180–1189.

──────; FERNANDEZ, C.; and MCAULIFFE, D. R. 1950. The excitatory process in the cochlea. *Proceedings of the National Academy of Science*, Washington, D.C. 36: 580–587.

References

DEUTSCH, L. J. 1968. The threshold of the stapedius reflex to selected acoustic stimuli in normal human ears. USN Submarine Medical Center Report No. 546: AD 685-774.

DJUPESLAND, G. 1962. Intra-aural muscular reflexes elicited by air current stimulation of the external ear. *Acta Otolaryngologica* 54: 143-153.

——— 1964. Middle ear muscle reflexes elicited by acoustic and nonacoustic stimulation. *Acta Otolaryngologica Supplement* 188: 287-292.

——— 1965. Electromyography of the tympanic muscles in man. *International Audiology* 4: 34-41.

ENGSTRÖM, H. 1967. The morphology of the normal sensory cells. *Acta Otolaryngologica* 63, appendix to nos. 2-3, p. 5-19.

———; ADES, H. W.; and ANDERSSON, A. 1966. *Structural pattern of the organ of Corti*. Baltimore: Williams and Wilkins.

FISCH, V., and VON SCHULTHESS, G. 1963. Electromyographic studies on the human stapedial muscle. *Acta Otolaryngologica* 56: 287-297.

FLETCHER, H. 1951. On the dynamics of the cochlea. *Journal of the Acoustical Society of America* 23: 637-645.

GERHARDT, H.-J.; DAVID, H., and MARX, I. 1966. Elektronenmikroskopische Untersuchungen am Musculus Tensor Tympani des Meerschweinchens. *Archiv für Klinische und Experimentelle Ohren-Nasen und Kehlkopfheilkunde* 186: 20-30.

GUINAN, J. J., JR., and PEAKE, W. T. 1967. Middle-ear characteristics of anesthetized cats. *Journal of the Acoustical Society of America* 41: 1237-1261.

HAMBERGER, C.-A., and WERSÄLL, J. 1964. Vascular supply of the tympanic membrane and the ossicular chain. *Acta Otolaryngologica Supplement* 188: 308-318.

HARRIS, J. D. 1972. A florilegium of 14 experiments in directional hearing. *Acta Otolaryngologica Supplement*.

HOLST, H.-E.; INGELSTEDT, S.; and ÖRTEGREN, U. 1963. Eardrum movements following stimulation of the middle-ear muscles. *Acta Otolaryngologica Supplement* 182: 73-93.

JOHNSTONE, J. R., and JOHNSTONE, B. M. 1965. Origin of summating potential. *Journal of the Acoustical Society of America* 40: 1405-1413.

KATAGIRI, S.; KAWAMOTO, K.; HORI, K.; and WATANUKI, K. 1968. Some surface views of the inner ear by light microscopy. *Acta Otolaryngologica* 66: 493-507.

KIANG, N. Y.-S., and PEAKE, W. T. 1960. Components of electrical responses recorded from the cochlea. *Annals of Otology, Rhinology, and Laryngology* 69: 448-458.

References

KIRIKAE, I. 1960. *The structure and function of the middle ear*. Toyko: University of Tokyo Press.

KLOCKHOFF, I. 1961. Middle-ear muscle reflexes in man. *Acta Otolaryngologica Supplement* 164.

―――, and ANDERSON, H. 1959. Recording of the stapedius reflex elicited by cutaneous stimulation. *Acta Otolaryngologica* 50: 451–454.

―――, and ANDERSON, H. 1960. Reflex activity in the tensor tympani muscle recorded in man. *Acta Otolaryngologica* 51: 184–188.

KOBRAK, H. G. 1948. Construction material of the sound conduction system of the human ear. *Journal of the Acoustical Society of America* 20: 125–130.

―――. 1959. *The Middle Ear*. Chicago: University of Chicago Press.

KONISHI, T.; KELSEY, ELIZABETH; and SINGLETON, G. T. 1967. Negative potential in scala media during early stage of anoxia. *Acta Otolaryngologica* 64: 107–118.

KRIEG, W. J. S. 1953. *Functional neuroanatomy*. Second ed., New York: Blakiston.

KUPPERMAN, R. 1966. The dynamic DC potential in the cochlea of the guinea pig (summating potential). *Acta Otolaryngologica* 62: 465–480.

LAWRENCE, M. 1962. The double innervation of the tensor tympani. *Annals of Otology, Rhinology, and Laryngology* 71: 705–718.

―――. 1967. Electric polarization of the tectorial membrane. *Annals of Otology, Rhinology, and Laryngology* 76: 287–312.

LEGOUIX, J. P. 1966. Observation des réponses microphoniques cochleares à des signaux de type impulsionnel. *Acustica* 16: 159–165.

LIDEN, G.; NORDLUND, B.; and HAWKINS, J. E., JR. 1963. Significance of the stapedius reflex for the understanding of speech. *Acta Otolaryngologica Supplement* 188: 275–279.

LINDSAY, J. R.; KOBRAK, H.; and PERLMAN, H. B. 1936. Relation of the stapedius reflex to hearing sensation in man. *Archives of Otolaryngology* 23: 671.

LOEB, M. 1964. Psychophysical correlates of intratympanic reflex action. *Psychological Bulletin* 61: 140–152.

―――, and FLETCHER, J. L. 1961. Contralateral threshold shift and reduction in temporary threshold shift as indices of acoustic reflex action. *Journal of the Acoustical Society of America* 33: 1558–1560.

―――, and RIOPELLE, A. J. 1960. Influence of loud contralateral stimulation on the threshold and perceived loudness of low-frequency tones. *Journal of the Acoustical Society of America* 32: 602–610.

Lowy, K. 1942. Cancellation of the electrical cochlear response with air- and bone-conducted sound. *Journal of the Acoustical Society of America* 14: 156–158.

Lüscher, E. 1929. Die Funktion des Musculus Stapedius beim Menschen. *Zentralblatt fuer Hals-usw. Heilk* 23: 105–132.

McArdle, Florence E., and Tonndorf, J. 1968. Perforations of the tympanic membrane and their effects upon middle-ear transmission. *Archiv für Klinische und Experimentelle Ohren-Nasen und Kehlkopfheilkunde* 192: 145–162.

Metz, O. 1946. The acoustic impedance measured on normal and pathological ears. *Acta Otolaryngologica Supplement* 63.

Møller, A. R. 1962. The sensitivity of contraction of the tympanic muscles in man. *Annals of Otology, Rhinology, and Laryngology* 71: 86–95.

———. 1965. An experimental study of the acoustic impedance of the middle ear and its transmission properties. *Acta Otolaryngologica* 60: 129–149.

Naftalin, L. 1967. The cochlear geometry as a frequency analyzer. *Journal of Laryngology and Otology* 81: 619–631.

———. 1968. Acoustic transmission and transduction in the peripheral hearing apparatus. *Progressive Biophysics* 18: 3–27.

Neergaard, E. B.; Anderson, H. C.; Hansen, C. C.; and Jepsen, O. 1963. Experimental studies on sound transmission in the human ear. III. Influence of the stapedius and tensor tympani muscles. *Acta Otolaryngologica Supplement* 188: 280–286.

Neergaard, E. B., and Rasmussen, P. E. 1966. Latency of the stapedius muscle reflex in man. *Archives of Otolaryngology* 84: 173–180.

Nordlund, B. 1962. Physical factors in sound localization. *Acta Otolaryngologica* 54: 75–93.

Onchi, Y. 1961. Mechanism of the middle ear. *Journal of the Acoustical Society of America* 33: 794–805.

Panayiotopoulos, C. P., and Stopp, Phyllis E. 1968. Effect of lithium and DNP on cochlear after-potential. *Journal of Physiology* (London) 197: 86–87P.

Perlman, H. B., and Case, T. J. 1939. Latent period of the crossed stapedius reflex in man. *Annals of Otology, Rhinology, and Laryngology* 48: 663–675.

Pichler, H., and Bornschein, H. 1957. Audiometrischer nachweis nichtakustisch ausgelöster reflexkontraktion der intraauralmuskulatur. *Acta Otolaryngologica* 48: 498–503.

Prather, W. F. 1961. Shifts in loudness of pure tones associated with contralateral noise stimulation. *Journal of Speech and Hearing Research* 4: 182–193.

References

Rawdon-Smith, A. F., and Hawkins, J. E., Jr. 1939. The electrical activity of a denervated ear. *Proceedings of the Royal Society of Medicine* 32: 496–507.

Reger, S. H.; Menzel, O. J.; Ickes, W. K.; and Steiner, S. J. 1963. Changes in air conduction and bone conduction sensitivity associated with voluntary contraction of middle-ear musculature. U.S. Army Medical Research Laboratory Report 576: 197–180.

Rubinstein, M.; Feldman, B.; Fischler, H.; Frei, E. H.; and Spira, D. 1966. Measurements of stapedial footplate displacements during transmission of sound through the middle ear. *Journal of the Acoustical Society of America* 40: 1420–1426.

Salomon, G., and Starr, A. 1963. Electromyography of middle-ear muscles in man during motor activities. *Acta Neurologica Scandinavica* 39: 161–168.

Schuknecht, H. 1960. Neuroanatomical correlates of auditory sensitivity and pitch discrimination in the cat. Ch. 6 in: *Neural Mechanisms of the Auditory and Vestibular Systems*, G. L. Rasmussen and W. F. Windle, eds. Springfield, Ill.: C. C. Thomas.

Sherrick, C. E., and Mangabeira-Albernaz, P. L. 1961. Auditory threshold shifts produced by simultaneously pulsed contra-lateral stimuli. *Journal of the Acoustical Society of America* 33: 1381–1385.

Sivian, L. J., and White, S. D. 1933. On minimum audible sound fields. *Journal of the Acoustical Society of America* 4: 288–321.

Spoendlin, H. 1966. *The organization of the cochlear receptor.* New York: S. Karger.

Stopp, P. E. 1967. "Afterpotential" in the cochlear response. *Nature* (London) 215: 1400.

Tasaki, I.; Davis, H.; and Eldredge, D. H. 1954. Exploration of cochlear potentials in guinea pig with a microelectrode. *Journal of the Acoustical Society of America* 26: 765–773.

Tasaki, I.; Davis, H.; and Legouix, J. P. 1952. The space-time pattern of the cochlear microphonics (guinea pig) as recorded by differential electrodes. *Journal of the Acoustical Society of America* 24: 502–519.

Tasaki, I., and Fernandez, C. 1952. Modifications of cochlear microphonics and action potential by KCl solution and by direct currents. *Journal of Neurophysiology* 15: 497–512.

Tasaki, I., and Spyropoulos, C. S. 1959. Stria vascularis as source of endocochlear potential. *Journal of Neurophysiology* 22: 149–155.

Teas, D. C.; Eldredge, D. H.; and Davis, H. 1962. Cochlear responses to acoustic transients: an interpretation of whole-nerve action potentials. *Journal of the Acoustical Society of America* 34: 1438–1459.

TERKILDSEN, K. 1960. Acoustic reflexes of the human musculus tensor tympani. *Acta Otolaryngologica Supplement* 158: 230–238.

TONNDORF, J., and KHANNA, S. M. 1967. Some properties of sound transmission in the middle and outer ears of cats. *Journal of the Acoustical Society of America* 41: 513–521.

———. 1970. The role of the tympanic membrane in middle-ear transmission. *Annals of Otology, Rhinology, and Laryngology* 79: 743–753.

TRUEX, R. C., and KELLNER, C. E. 1948. *Detailed atlas of the head and neck.* New York: Oxford University Press.

WEISS, H. S.; MUNDIE, J. R.; CASHIN, J. L.; and SHINABARGER, E. W. 1962. The normal human intra-aural muscle reflex in response to sound. *Acta Otolaryngologica* 55: 505–515.

WEVER, E. G. 1949. *Theories of hearing.* New York: Wiley.

———, and BRAY, C. W. 1937. The effects of chemical substances upon the electrical responses of the cochlea: I. The application of sodium chloride to the round window membrane. *Annals of Otology, Rhinology, and Laryngology* 46: 291–302.

———, and LAWRENCE, M. 1952. The place principle in auditory theory. *Proceedings of the National Academy of Science,* Washington, D.C. 38: 133–138.

———, and LAWRENCE, M. 1954. *Physiological acoustics.* Princeton, N.J.: Princeton University Press.

———; LAWRENCE, M.; and SMITH, K. R. 1948. The middle ear in sound conduction. *Archives of Otolaryngology* 48: 19–35.

WHITFIELD, I. C., and ROSS, H. F. 1965. Cochlear-microphonic and summating potentials and the outputs of individual hair-cell generators. *Journal of the Acoustical Society of America* 38: 126–131.

WIENER, F. M. 1947. On the diffraction of a progressive sound wave by the human head. *Journal of the Acoustical Society of America* 19: 143–146.

———, and ROSS, D. A. 1946. The pressure distribution in the auditory canal in a progressive sound field. *Journal of the Acoustical Society of America* 18: 401–408.

SUGGESTED READINGS

DAVIS, H. 1970. Anatomy and physiology of the auditory system. *Hearing and Deafness*, H. Davis and S. R. Silverman, eds. Third edition. New York: Holt, Rinehart and Winston. Pp. 47–63.

Admirably pitched to the beginner in audiology by the master in this field.

FLETCHER, S. G. 1970. The hearing mechanism. *The hard of hearing child*, F. S. Berg and S. G. Fletcher, eds. New York: Grune and Stratton. Pp. 29–40.

Brief, but not outdated hopelessly as so many other 10-page surveys are.

GULICK, W. L. 1971. *Hearing*. New York: Oxford University Press. Pp. 27–41, 52–68.

Appropriate introductory material to the mechanisms of the peripheral ear.

LITTLER, T. S. 1965. *The physics of the ear*. New York: Pergamon Press. Pp. 1–9, 22–37, 62–88.

Excellent material, though not for beginners; perhaps for second-year students of hearing science.

STEVENS, S. S., and WARSHOFSKY, F. 1965. *Sound and hearing*. New York: Time, Inc.

Slick, beautifully illustrated, although somewhat over-simplified.

THOMPSON, R. F. 1967. *Foundations of physiological psychology*. New York: Harper and Row. Pp. 261–66.

Recent succinct material for the sensory psychologist.

TOWE, A. L. 1966. *Physiology and biophysics*, T. C. Ruch and H. D. Patton, eds. Philadelphia: W. B. Saunders.

Good coverage for the physiologically minded.

WHITFIELD, I. C. 1967. *The auditory pathway*. Baltimore: Williams and Wilkins. Pp. 14–52.

Clear but rather advanced for the beginner in audiology. Excellent treatment for students in experimental/physiological psychology or physiology.